SBAs and EMQs for the MRCOG Part 2

SBAs and EMQs for the MRCOG Part 2

Second edition

Edited by

Sai Gnanasambanthan
Speciality Trainee (ST7) in Obstetrics and Gynaecology,
Princess Royal University Hospital, King's College NHS Trust, London, UK

Shreelata T. Datta
Consultant Obstetrician and Gynaecologist,
East Sussex Healthcare NHS Trust, Sussex, UK

Tahir Mahmood
Consultant Obstetrician and Gynaecologist
Victoria Hospital, Kirkcaldy,
Fife and Spire Murrayfield Hospital, Edinburgh, UK

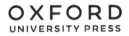

OXFORD
UNIVERSITY PRESS

OXFORD
UNIVERSITY PRESS

Great Clarendon Street, Oxford, OX2 6DP,
United Kingdom

Oxford University Press is a department of the University of Oxford.
It furthers the University's objective of excellence in research, scholarship,
and education by publishing worldwide. Oxford is a registered trade mark of
Oxford University Press in the UK and in certain other countries

First Edition published in 2018
Second Edition published in 2024

Published in the United States of America by Oxford University Press
198 Madison Avenue, New York, NY 10016, United States of America

British Library Cataloguing in Publication Data
Data available

Library of Congress Control Number: 2023952634

ISBN 978–0–19–888845–1

DOI: 10.1093/med/9780198888451.001.0001

Printed in the UK by
Ashford Colour Press Ltd, Gosport, Hampshire

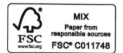

MIX
Paper from
responsible sources
FSC® C011748

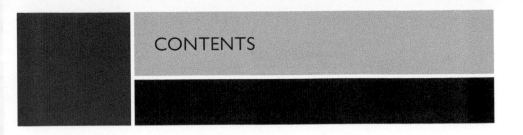

CONTENTS

Paper 6

ABOUT THE EDITORS

Sai Gnanasambanthan is a South London final year Speciality Trainee in Obstetrics and Gynaecology. Her interests lie in maternal medicine and intrapartum care, and she has a passion for multiprofessional training and quality improvement of care for pregnant patients with diabetes. She has completed her postgraduate certificate in Medical Education with Merit. She is involved in teaching and mentoring doctors planning to sit the MRCOG examinations.

Shreelata T. Datta is a Consultant Obstetrician and Gynaecologist with a special interest in benign gynaecology, colposcopy, and ultrasound. She was awarded the RCOG Edgar Gentilli Prize and the BMA Helen Lawson award for her research in ovarian cancer. She has a passion for teaching, having obtained a Master's in Clinical Education with Merit and was appointed Associate Clinical Dean at King's College Medical School.

Tahir Mahmood has worked as Consultant Obstetrician and Gynaecologist NHS Fife since 1990, has served as Vice President Standards Royal College of Obstetricians and Gynaecologist, UK (RCOG), and as President European Board and College of Obstetrics and Gynaecology (EBCOG). Currently he chairs the Quality Assurance Committee of the EBCOG Examination for European Fellowships in Obstetrics and Gynaecology.

HOW TO APPROACH THE EXAM

From March 2015, the format of the MRCOG Part 2 consists of two parts, each of which count for 50% of the total score. In each paper there are two question formats: 50 single best answer questions (SBAs) and 50 extended matching questions (EMQs). The duration of each exam is three hours, with no formal time allocation to each section. However, the RCOG recommends spending 110 minutes on the EMQ paper and 70 minutes on the SBA paper, given that the EMQ component carries 60% of the total mark. The RCOG website, https://www.rcog.org.uk, provides further detail on the exam format, together with some sample questions, which you should be familiar with.

In the months leading up to the exam, make sure you are up-to-date with all clinical guidelines and practice in the UK. This includes familiarizing yourself with the RCOG Green-top Guidelines, patient information forms, consent advice, and scientific advisory papers. Non-RCOG guidance which you should refer to include the CEMACH/CEMACE reports, NICE Guidelines, *The Obstetrician and Gynaecologist*, *A Guide to the Part 2 MRCOG* and the *MRCOG and Beyond* series. A useful website is https://elearning.rcog.org.uk.

Three or four months before the exam, you should start developing exam technique by practising exam papers. This will develop your ability to time-keep in an exam setting. Practising exam papers will also provide insight into whether you need to allocate more time to EMQs or SBAs. It may help to understand the structure of the questions. EMQs have four components: the theme, answer options, the instructions, and the question items. SBAs, on the other hand, consist simply of a question and five answer options. Some SBAs include a lead-in statement preceding the question. In both SBAs and EMQs, the answer options are in alphabetical or in some other logical order.

When in the exam, be sure to read each question and its parts carefully, perhaps highlighting or underlining important points. Try to come to the answer *before* looking at the options available. To answer a question correctly, you must have a clear concept of the topic, along with in-depth knowledge of the clinical area. If the answer option has multiple parts, make sure that all parts are correct in relation to the question item before selecting it as the correct answer. Try to focus on what you would do if you encountered each scenario in real life, perhaps in the clinic or on the labour ward.

Finally, it is important to remember that each correct answer is awarded one mark. Incorrect answers are not penalized, so it is in your interest to answer every question. Allocate some time to ensure the answer sheet is correctly filled in.

Good luck!

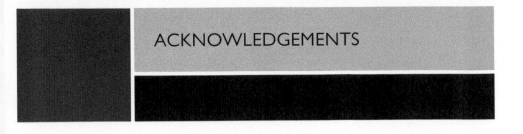

ACKNOWLEDGEMENTS

We would like to acknowledge the question writers and reviewers for the first edition who produced questions as part of an online project for OUP. These questions are included in this book.

Christina Aye

Kalsang Bhatia

Timothy Bracewell-Milnes

Gail Fullerton

Charity Khoo

Edward Morris

Rachel O'Donnell

Nithiya Palaniappan

Saurabh Phadnis

Karin Piegsa

ABBREVIATIONS

ABC	Airway, breathing, circulation
ACE	angiotensin-converting enzyme
AFC	Antral follicle count
AFI	Amniotic fluid index
AMH	Anti-Müllerian hormone
APS	Antiphospholipid syndrome
ARCP	Annual Review of Competency Progression
ARDS	Acute respiratory disease syndrome
ARM	Artificial rupture of the amniotic membranes
BBV	Blood-borne virus
BC	Birth centre
BCG	Bacille Calmette–Guerin vaccination for TB
BMI	Body mass index
BSO	Bilateral salpingoophorectomy
BV	Bacterial vaginosis
CAH	Congenital adrenal hyperplasia
CCT	Certification of completion of training
CEU	Clinical Effectiveness Unit
CHC	Combined hormonal contraception
CIN	Cervical intraepithelial neoplasia
CMACE	Centre for Maternal and Child Enquiries
CMV	Cytomegalovirus
CNS	Central nervous system
CO	Cardiac output
COC	Combined oral contraception
COCP	Combined oral contraceptive pill
CPVP	Chronic post-vasectomy pain
CS	Caesarean section
CTG	Cardiotocography
CTP	Combined transdermal patch
CTPA	CT pulmonary angiogram

CVR	Combined vaginal ring
CVS	Chorionic villus sampling
DCDA	Dichorionic diamniotic
DOA	Direct occiput anterior
DOPS	Direct observation of physical skill
DVT	Deep vein thrombosis
EC	Emergency contraception
ECV	External cephalic version
EE	Ethinylestradiol
FASP	Foetal Anomaly Screening Programme
FFP	Fresh frozen plasma
FGM	Female genital mutilation
FIGO	The International Federation of Gynecology and Obstetrics
FISH	Fluorescence in situ hybridization
FSH	Follicle stimulating hormone
FSRH	Faculty of Sexual & Reproductive Health
GBS	Group B streptococcus
GBS	Group B streptococcus
GDM	Gestational diabetes mellitus
GMC	General Medical Council
GnRH	Gonadotropin-releasing hormone
GTD	Gestational trophoblastic disease
GTN	Gestational trophoblastic neoplasia
GTN	Glyceryl trinitrate
GTT	Glucose tolerance test
HAART	Highly active antiretroviral therapy
HCG	Human chorionic gonadotropin
HDL	High-density lipoprotein
HMB	Heavy menstrual bleeding
HPV	Human papilloma virus
HR	Heart rate
HRT	Hormone replacement therapy
HSDD	Hypoactive sexual desire disorder
HSV	Herpes simplex virus
ICSI	Intracytoplasmic sperm injection
IOL	Induction of labour
IOTA	International Ovarian Tumour Analysis
ITU	Intensive therapy unit
IUCD	Intrauterine copper device

IUD	Intrauterine death
IUD	Intrauterine device
IUGR	Intrauterine growth restriction
IUI	Intrauterine insemination
IUS	Intrauterine system
IVF	In-vitro fertilization
JVP	Jugular venous pressure
LFT	Liver function tests
LH	Luteinizing hormone
LLETZ	Large loop excision of the transformation zone
LMWH	Low-molecular-weight heparin
LOA	Left occiput anterior
LOT	Left occiput transverse
LP	Lichen planus
MCDA	Monochorionic diamniotic
MCMA	Monochorionic monoamniotic
MMR	Measles, mumps, and rubella
MRSA	Methicillin-resistant *Staphylococcus aureus*
MSU	Midstream specimen of urine
NEWS	National Early Warning Score
NNRTI	Non-nucleoside reverse transcriptase inhibitors
NRTI	Nucleoside reverse transcriptase inhibitors
NSAID	Non-steroidal anti-inflammatory drug
OC	Obstetric cholestasis
OGTT	Oral glucose tolerance test
OHSS	Ovarian hyperstimulation syndrome
OPG	Office of the public guardian
OSATS	Objective structured assessment of technical skills
OSCE	Objective structured clinical examination
PCOS	Polycystic ovary syndrome
PE	Pulmonary embolism
PEA	Pulseless electrical activity
PEPSE	Post-exposure prophylaxis after sexual exposure
PET	Pre-eclampsia toxaemia
PI	Protease inhibitors
POC	Posterior circulation syndrome
POP	Progestogen-only pill
PPH	Post-partum haemorrhage
PPROM	Preterm prelabour rupture of membranes

PPV	Positive predictive value
PUL	Pregnancy of unknown location
RMI	Risk of malignancy index
RNA	Ribonucleic acid
SERM	Selective oestrogen receptor modulator
SHBG	Sex hormone binding globulin
SHO	Senior house officer
SIDS	Sudden infant death syndrome
SLE	Systemic lupus erythematosus
SPC	Summary of product characteristics
SROM	Spontaneous rupture of membrane
SSRI	Selective serotonin reuptake inhibitor
STEMI	ST-elevation myocardial infarction
STI	Sexually transmitted infection
SV	Stroke volume
TAH	Total abdominal hysterectomy
TB	Tuberculosis
TOT	Transobturator tape
TSH	Thyroid-stimulating hormone
TTTS	Twin transfusion syndrome
TVT	Tension-free vaginal tape
TVUS	Transvaginal ultrasound scan
UAE	Uterine arterial embolization
UKMEC	UK Medical Eligibility Criteria
USS	Ultrasound scan
VaIN	Vaginal intraepithelial neoplasia
VBAC	Vaginal birth after caesarean
VIN	Vulval intraepithelial neoplasia
VTE	Venous thromboembolism
VZIG	Varicella zoster immunoglobulin
VZV	Varicella zoster virus

CONTRIBUTORS TO THE FIRST EDITION

Dr Ibrahim Alsharaydeh

Mr Jayanta Chatterjee

Dr Gomathy Gopal

Dr Timothy Hookway

Dr Aravind Subramaniam

INTRODUCTION

Obtaining the membership of the Royal College of Obstetricians and Gynaecologists (RCOG) is a core part of training to become a specialist in obstetrics and gynaecology in the UK and in many other countries. To become a member of the RCOG, one must pass a knowledge-based exam, which requires the clinical application of theoretical knowledge. In 2015 the format of the exam was altered. It comprises two papers, each three hours in duration, incorporating 50 single best answer questions (SBAs), worth 40% of the total mark, and 50 extended matching questions (EMQs), worth 60% of the total mark. The method of assessment has recently changed from written to computer-based testing, but the format remains the same. Approximately 20–30% of all candidates pass this part of the exam and go on to sit the OSCE component of the exam.

The aim of this book is not to provide another revision text to consult, but rather to tackle the common and difficult areas faced by candidates undertaking the exam. Questions have been compiled by junior doctors who have recently passed the exam, together with consultants who have a special interest in postgraduate education and training. The structure and content of the book matches the format of the exam. A detailed explanation is provided along with each answer, as well as appropriate references where relevant. Whilst this book is focused on the UK MRCOG Part 2 exam, it will also be useful for candidates anywhere in the world who are attempting postgraduate examinations in this speciality, wherever a similar format is applied.

We have reviewed each paper to ensure that all key areas outlined in the *MRCOG Syllabus and Knowledge Requirements for Core Curriculum 2019* are covered in this book. However, we understand that omissions do occur and therefore would welcome feedback at mrcog2@gmail.com. All that remains for us to do is to wish you the very best of luck in passing the computer-based component of the MRCOG Part 2 exam.

Sai Gnanasambanthan
Shreelata Datta
Tahir Mahmood
July 2023

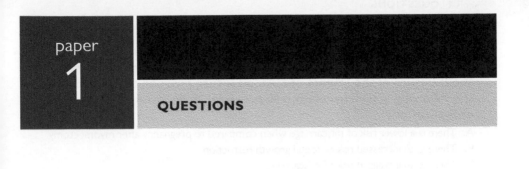

Single Best Answers

1. You are asked to see a pregnant woman who has been referred for a chest X-ray for suspected pneumonia at 24 weeks gestation. She is worried about the impact of exposure to ionizing radiation on her pregnancy. What is the accepted cumulative dose of ionizing radiation in pregnancy?

   A. 50 mGy
   B. 100 mGy
   C. 150 mGy
   D. 250 mGy
   E. 500 mGy

2. You review a patient who is going to start brachytherapy for cervical cancer. She is worried about the impact of radiotherapy on her vagina. What is the reported rate of dyspareunia after radiotherapy for cervical carcinoma?

   A. 10%
   B. 20%
   C. 35%
   D. 50%
   E. 65%

3. You are asked to see a 36-year-old multiparous woman who is keen
    to proceed with a uterine artery embolization for fibroids. However,
    she is unsure of the impact of UAE on future pregnancies. Which of
    the following is true in relation to pregnancies following uterine artery
    embolization?

    A. There is a lower risk of miscarriage when compared to pregnancy after myomectomy
    B. There is an increased risk of foetal growth restriction
    C. There is an increased risk of miscarriage
    D. There is an increased risk of preterm delivery
    E. There is no increase in the rate of caesarean section

4. A 34-year-old woman has consented for a surgical evacuation of the
    uterus for early pregnancy loss. Which of the following is a serious risk?

    A. Localized pelvic infection
    B. Repeat surgical evacuation, up to 5 in 100 women
    C. Significant trauma to the cervix
    D. Uterine perforation, up to 10 in 1,000 women
    E. Vaginal bleeding lasting up to two weeks after the procedure

5. A 42-year-old woman has lost two litres of blood at emergency
    caesarean section for foetal distress (DCDA twins). When considering
    the administration of blood and blood products, which of the following
    is correct?

    A. Fresh frozen plasma (FFP) contains more fibrinogen than cryoprecipitate
    B. FFP is derived from whole blood and does not contain clotting factors
    C. FFP is stored at −30 °C and needs to be defrosted thoroughly prior to administration
    D. A prothrombin time and activated partial thromboplastin time ratio below 1.5 is associated
       with an increased risk of a clinical coagulopathy
    E. A unit of concentrated red cells increases the haematocrit by 8%

6. You review a 26-year-old epileptic woman on the postnatal ward
    following a ventouse delivery and second-degree tear. She is taking
    lamotrigine and is keen to breastfeed. Her last fit was two months prior
    to pregnancy. What advice would you give her?

    A. Administer 1 mg intravenous vitamin K to the neonate
    B. Avoid breastfeeding if possible
    C. Consider breastfeeding prior to taking lamotrigine
    D. Stop anti-epileptic medication
    E. Stop lamotrigine and commence carbamazepine

7. **A 23-year-old primiparous woman has been diagnosed with pulmonary tuberculosis at 33 weeks gestation. What is the impact on the pregnancy?**
    A. Increased risk of congenital anomaly
    B. Increased risk of placental abruption
    C. Increased risk of pneumonia
    D. Increased risk of pre-eclampsia
    E. Increased risk of preterm rupture of membranes

8. **A 34-year-old woman attends your clinic for long-term contraception. She is not keen on hormonal therapy, but is interested in the intrauterine copper device (IUCD). Which of the following is a risk associated with the IUCD?**
    A. The IUCD cannot be used in women with HIV
    B. The IUCD is associated with heavier menstrual bleeding and intermenstrual spotting
    C. The IUCD should be removed in women with asymptomatic *Actinomyces*-like organisms
    D. There is a higher risk of ectopic pregnancy
    E. There is a higher risk of infertility

9. **You prescribe cyproterone acetate to a 28-year-old woman presenting with simple hirsutism. What type of medication is cyproterone acetate?**
    A. Aldosterone antagonist
    B. Anti-oestrogen
    C. Diuretic
    D. Oestrogen receptor agonist
    E. Progestogen

10. **A 25-year-old primigravid woman presents in her first trimester. You note from her blood results that she is hyperthyroid. Which of the following is correct regarding her medication?**
    A. Carbimazole is preferred to propylthiouracil
    B. Foetal thyroxine levels may be affected
    C. The risk of agranulocytosis is lower with carbimazole than propylthiouracil
    D. Treatment doses will need to be increased later in pregnancy
    E. When hyperthyroidism is seen with hyperemesis gravidarum, antithyroid drugs should be given

11. **A 46-year-old nulliparous woman is seen with bloating and weight loss. Ultrasound confirms the presence of an irregular vascular 7 cm solid lesion adjacent to the left ovary. Ascites is present. What is the most appropriate course of management?**
    A. Abdominal hysterectomy, bilateral salpingo-oophorectomy, and omental biopsy
    B. Laparoscopic removal of left ovarian mass
    C. Laparotomy and removal of left ovarian mass
    D. Refer to gynaecology oncologist
    E. Request MRI pelvis

12. **You are asked to see a 32-year-old nulliparous woman and her 34-year-old husband in an infertility clinic. They are both fit and healthy and have been trying to conceive for almost two years. On reviewing the laboratory investigations of the semen analysis, you find that the sperm count is <2×10⁶/ml in two separate samples. All other parameters are normal, as are the FSH, LH, and testosterone. What is the most likely cause?**
    A. Congenital absence of the vas deferens
    B. Kallmann syndrome
    C. Paternal age
    D. Primary testicular failure
    E. Varicocele

13. **You see a 34-year-old woman in the recurrent miscarriage clinic. She is fit and well, and cytogenetic analysis of the products of conception for her third miscarriage was normal. Which blood investigation would you request first?**
    A. Blood glucose level
    B. Free T4 and TSH levels
    C. Lupus anticoagulant
    D. Parental karyotype
    E. Pelvic ultrasound

14. **You are asked to review the blood investigations of a primiparous woman who is 22 weeks pregnant. You notice she has an isolated raised inhibin A level. What complication is associated with a high inhibin A level?**
    A. Oligohydramnios
    B. Placental abruption
    C. Pre-eclampsia
    D. Spontaneous miscarriage
    E. Trisomy 21

15. **You are asked to audit the triggers for incident reporting in maternity. Which of the following are trigger factors for incident reporting?**
    A. A baby born with Apgar score less than 5 at one minute
    B. An estimated blood loss over 1,000 ml at delivery
    C. A stillbirth less than 450 g
    D. A term baby admitted to the neonatal unit
    E. Vaginal breech delivery

16. **Caesarean section (CS) is associated with which of the following risks:**
    A. A 1-in-1,000 risk of bladder injury requiring repair
    B. After their first CS, 1 in 1,000 women will have an increased risk of placenta praevia or placenta accreta
    C. An increase by 10% of the overall risk profile with emergency CS when compared to elective CS
    D. No increased risk of stillbirth in future pregnancies
    E. Neonatal lacerations in 0.1% of caesareans

17. **A 13-year-old girl alleges rape by a neighbour six weeks ago. She does not use tampons and states that she has never had sexual intercourse prior to that incident. Which of the following genital findings support the allegation of vaginal penetration?**
    A. Annular hymen
    B. Crescentic hymen
    C. Cribriform hymen
    D. Fimbriated hymen
    E. Transected hymen

18. **A 32-year-old woman contemplating her first pregnancy comes to see you in the pre-pregnancy clinic. She has had epilepsy since the age of 10. Which of the following are true about anticonvulsants in pregnancy:**
    A. Clonazepam is teratogenic
    B. Phenobarbitone and carbamazepine crosses the placenta
    C. Phenytoin is not associated with congenital heart defects
    D. Primidone does not cross the placenta
    E. The teratogenic risk of a combined anticonvulsant regime, which includes valproate, carbamazepine, and phenytoin, is as high as 10%

19. **A woman who is Rhesus-negative undergoes a laparoscopic salpingectomy for an ectopic pregnancy at eight weeks gestation. What dose of anti-D immunoglobulin should she receive immediately after the operation?**
    A. 250 IU
    B. 500 IU
    C. 1,000 IU
    D. 1,500 IU
    E. Anti-D is not necessary as she is in the first trimester of pregnancy

20. **The cardiovascular system undergoes numerous changes in pregnancy to adapt to the demands of the developing foetus and labour. Which of the following parameters does not change?**
    A. Blood volume
    B. Capillary refill time
    C. Cardiac output
    D. Heart rate
    E. Stroke volume

21. **A 26-year-old woman with known endometriosis would like to try the Mirena coil. What is the most common risk associated with the Mirena coil?**
    A. Expulsion, occurring in 1% of cases
    B. Expulsion, occurring in 5% of cases
    C. Failed contraception, occurring in 1% of cases
    D. Perforation, occurring in 1% of cases
    E. Perforation, occurring in 5% of cases

22. **A 30-year-old woman presents at 28 weeks gestation in her second pregnancy. She is known to have anti-C antibodies. On reviewing her latest blood results, you notice that her anti-C titre is 27 IU/ml. How would you manage her?**
    A. Continue to monitor anti-C levels every two weeks
    B. Refer to a specialist unit for amniocentesis
    C. Refer to specialist unit for an ultrasound to measure the middle cerebral peak systolic velocity
    D. Refer to a specialist unit for an ultrasound to measure the umbilical artery Doppler
    E. Repeat anti-C levels in one week

23. **A 39-year-old primiparous woman visits her sister and nephew. Five days later, her nephew develops symptoms associated with rubella infection. What is the incubation period for rubella?**
    A. 5 days
    B. 7 days
    C. 10 days
    D. 14 days
    E. 25 days

24. **You review a 22-year-old woman admitted with severe OHSS. What is your management plan?**
    A. Commence intravenous antibiotics
    B. Commence vigorous intravenous crystalloid therapy
    C. Perform an ascitic tap if oliguric
    D. Prescribe dopamine agonists
    E. Prescribe thromboprophylaxis

25. **A 33-year-old woman presents to your clinic. Her mother and aunt have had breast cancer and she has been found to be a carrier of the *BRCA1* mutation. What is the impact of the *BRCA1* mutation on ovarian cancer?**

    A. *BRCA* mutation carriers are likely to present at an earlier stage of ovarian cancer
    B. *BRCA* mutation carriers have a better prognosis for ovarian cancer than non-carriers
    C. The estimated risk of ovarian cancer is 20% in *BRCA1* mutation carriers
    D. The grade of ovarian cancer is the same in *BRCA* mutation carriers as it is for the general population
    E. Tumours in *BRCA* carriers are more likely to be granulosa cell tumours

26. **A 34-year-old primigravid woman presents at 32 weeks gestation with shortness of breath and abdominal pain. On palpation, her abdomen appears tense and large for dates. It is difficult to establish presentation and an ultrasound confirms polyhydramnios. Which of the following is a cause for polyhydramnios?**

    A. Carbamazepine treatment for epilepsy
    B. Maternal diabetes insipidus
    C. Placental chorioangioma
    D. Trisomy 18
    E. Twin pregnancy

27. **In post-partum haemorrhage (PPH), which of the following is correct?**

    A. A blood loss of over 40% of total blood volume of a 70-kg woman is considered 'life-threatening'
    B. During CS, it is routine practice to administer a slow intravenous dose of 10 IU of oxytocin as a prophylactic measure to reduce the risk of PPH
    C. Ergometrine is absolutely contraindicated in management of severe PPH in a woman who is known to have had hypertension in pregnancy
    D. Misoprostol has been shown to be as effective as oxytocin in the management of post-partum haemorrhage
    E. Prophylactic oxytocics given routinely in the management of the third stage of labour reduce the risk of PPH in more than 90% of cases

28. **A 34-year-old woman with an IVF pregnancy attends the foetal medicine unit for selective embryo reduction. Which of the following is correct?**

    A. There is a 20% risk of miscarriage
    B. There is a higher risk of miscarriage in subsequent pregnancies
    C. There is an increase in short-term mortality of the remaining twin
    D. There is an increase in long-term morbidity of the remaining twin
    E. There is a risk of significant regret

29. **A 40-year-old woman presents at 12 weeks gestation in her second pregnancy. Her first child has trisomy 21 and she is keen to proceed with invasive embryo testing. Which of the following is correct?**
    A. Amniocentesis is usually performed at 13 weeks gestation
    B. CVS can be performed from nine weeks gestation
    C. The risk of miscarriage associated with CVS is 1%
    D. There is a 2% culture failure rate with amniocentesis
    E. The use of FISH reduces the delay in obtaining a result for amniocentesis

30. **A representative from the pharmacy team would like to introduce you to a new progestogen on the hospital formulary. Which of the following is true?**
    A. Progestogens are effective in treating ovulatory dysfunctional uterine bleeding
    B. Progestogens are effective in treating premenstrual symptoms
    C. Progestogens are less effective than NSAIDs and antifibrinolytics in anovulatory menorrhagia
    D. Progestogens can be used to treat metropathia haemorrhagica
    E. Progestogens should be used continuously for up to five days to stop bleeding

31. **A 25-year-old woman who is known to have beta thalassaemia trait is due to marry someone from the same ethnic background. Which of the following is correct?**
    A. If her fiancé is screen positive, there is a 50% chance that the foetus will suffer from beta thalassaemia major
    B. Parenteral iron can be used for treatment
    C. She will not suffer from anaemia
    D. Thalassaemia major is associated with cardiac failure
    E. Thalassaemia major is not life-threatening

32. **Upon attending an emergency buzzer call-out on the labour ward, you find a woman with cord prolapse. Which one of the following is a risk factor for umbilical cord prolapse?**
    A. 3 cm fundal subserosal fibroid
    B. Meconium liquor
    C. Placenta praevia
    D. Primigravid woman
    E. Transverse presentation

33. **You are reviewing a 36-year-old woman who has undergone a surgical evacuation for a molar pregnancy. Which one of the following forms part of the FIGO scoring system for gestational trophoblastic disease (GTD)?**
    A. Heavy bleeding at the time of surgical evacuation
    B. Parity
    C. Pregnancy gestation
    D. Previous history of childhood malignancy
    E. Tumour size

34. **A 24-year-old woman presents with a mild fever, feeling unwell with joint pain. She is 36 weeks pregnant and diagnosed to have human parvovirus B19 infection. What is the rate of vertical transmission at this gestation?**
    A. 10%
    B. 20%
    C. 30%
    D. 50%
    E. 70%

35. **A 56-year-old postmenopausal woman is referred to clinic with a six-month history of bloating. Ultrasound reveals a 7 cm multilocular unilateral ovarian cyst with solid areas. There is no ascites. CA125 is 55. What is her RMI?**
    A. 110
    B. 220
    C. 330
    D. 440
    E. 500

36. **You are asked to review the ultrasound results for a 42-year-old primigravid woman at 12 weeks gestation. The result suggests a high risk of trisomy 21. Which of the following is correct regarding the aetiology of trisomy 21?**
    A. 10% of babies with Down's syndrome are born with cardiac anomalies
    B. About 45% of cases are due to meiotic non-disjunction
    C. After two affected foetuses the recurrence rate is almost 30%
    D. If the father carries a Robertsonian translocation affecting chromosome 21, the recurrence risk is 10%
    E. Recurrence rate is affected by maternal age

37. **A 35-year-old woman presents with non-specific abdominal pain; ultrasound scan showed a 5-mm echogenic focus polyp in the uterine cavity. Both ovaries appear normal. She has normal regular withdrawal bleeding with the combined oral contraceptive pill and tells you her pain has resolved with the pill. What would your management plan be?**
    A. Endometrial biopsy
    B. Follow-up hysteroscopy in six months to assess any change
    C. Hysteroscopic resection of the polyp
    D. Reassure and discharge to GP
    E. Repeat ultrasound in six months

38. During investigation of lower urinary tract symptoms, videourodynamics would be preferred to conventional urodynamics in which of the following scenarios?

A. Clinical suspicion of detrusor overactivity
B. Mixed symptoms (frequency, urgency, and stress incontinence)
C. Previously unsuccessful incontinence surgery
D. Symptoms unresponsive to conservative therapy
E. Voiding difficulties

39. You see an anxious 26-year-old primigravid woman in an antenatal clinic. She asks you about the benefits of breastfeeding. Which of the following is correct?

A. Breastfeeding should be initiated within three hours of birth to maximize success
B. Colostrum has high levels of carbohydrate
C. Colostrum is especially rich in IgE
D. Colostrum is produced in small quantities after the birth of the baby
E. In the UK, about 10% of mothers are still breastfeeding at six months

40. A 35-year-old woman is diagnosed with hypothalamic hypogonadism. She would like to conceive. What treatment would you administer to stimulate ovulation?

A. Clomiphene
B. Gonadotrophin therapy
C. Metformin
D. Ovarian drilling
E. Pulsatile gonadotrophin-releasing hormone

41. A 36-year-old woman presents after being exposed to a five-year-old child who develops chickenpox. She cannot remember having chickenpox. Which of the following is correct?

A. More than 90% of the UK antenatal population are seropositive for varicella zoster IgG
B. Pneumonia occurs in up to 20% of pregnant women with chickenpox
C. The risk of spontaneous miscarriage is increased if chickenpox occurs in the first trimester
D. Routine immunization to varicella is advised in pregnancy
E. Varicella zoster immunoglobulin should be given as soon as clinical signs of chickenpox have developed

42. **An emergency CS was performed on a 25-year-old woman for worsening pre-eclampsia with failed induction of labour at 36 weeks gestation. Four hours after the CS, her blood pressure was 180/95 mmHg, and her urine output around 15 ml/hour. What is your management plan?**

    A. Administer a loading dose of 1 g magnesium sulphate followed by infusion
    B. Administer an immediate fluid challenge
    C. Administer intravenous frusemide 10–20 mg
    D. Prescribe intravenous antihypertensive treatment
    E. Prescribe oral antihypertensive treatment

43. **A 34-year-old woman in her second pregnancy presents with a one-day history of headache and vomiting at 24 weeks gestation. She describes the headache as being on the left side only, pulsating, and severe in intensity. She is unable to perform her activities of daily living, as this aggravates the pain. Lying in a dark room limits the pain. All observations and examination are normal. What is the diagnosis?**

    A. Cerebral venous thrombosis
    B. Idiopathic intracranial hypertension
    C. Migraine
    D. Pituitary tumour
    E. Subarachnoid haemorrhage

44. **You are asked to review a 22-year-old woman in her first pregnancy because she has type 4 female genital mutilation. Which of the following does this include?**

    A. Genital piercing
    B   Infibulation
    C. Partial removal of the clitoris
    D. Removal of the clitoris and prepuce
    E. Total removal of the clitoris

45. **When counselling a recently postmenopausal woman with unpleasant vasomotor symptoms wishing to take hormone replacement therapy (HRT), it is important to discuss fully the risks and benefits of HRT. Which one of the following statements should be part of the discussion:**

    A. No protection of lower genital tract symptoms
    B. No increase in the risk of venous thromboembolic disease
    C. Increased risk of painless vertebral osteoporotic fracture
    D. Protection from Alzheimer's disease
    E. Increased risk of colonic cancer

46. **A 28-year-old hyperthyroid woman with a 6 cm left ovarian mass undergoes a left salpingo-oophorectomy. Following the operation, she experiences symptoms of hypothyroidism and consequently is recommended to stop her antithyroid medication. What type of ovarian tumour does she have?**
    A. Brenner's tumour
    B. Granulosa cell tumour
    C. Immature malignant teratoma
    D. Sertoli–Leydig tumour
    E. Struma ovarii

47. **A 57-year-old woman who has had two children presents with the sensation of 'something coming down' with no urinary symptoms. She complains of chronic constipation. On examination, she has stage 2–3 posterior vaginal wall prolapse with no associated uterine descent. The anterior vaginal wall is well supported. What is the most appropriate treatment?**
    A. Paravaginal wall repair
    B. Pelvic floor exercises
    C. Posterior vaginal wall repair
    D. Posterior vaginal wall repair with mesh
    E. Shelf pessary

48. **A 24-year-old nulliparous woman presents with headaches and milky discharge from her breasts. She also complains of vomiting, for which she is taking medication. What is the most likely physiological cause?**
    A. Breastfeeding
    B. Caesarean section
    C. Chronic renal failure
    D. Metoclopramide
    E. PCOS

49. **Which of the following has an association with endometrial cancer?**
    A. Bilateral salpingo-oophorectomy (BSO)
    B. *BRCA2*
    C. Granulosa cell tumours
    D. HER-2 receptor agonist
    E. High SHBG (sex hormone binding globulin)

50. **You review a 65-year-old woman with known urinary urgency and prescribe oxybutynin. Which class of drug is this?**
    A. Antimuscarinic
    B. Calcium channel inhibitor
    C. Cox inhibitor
    D. Dopamine agonist
    E. Loop diuretic

Extended Matching Questions

Options for questions 1–5

For each of the following clinical scenarios, choose the single diagnosis or most appropriate treatment. Each option may be used once, more than once, or not at all.

   A. Cerebral vascular thrombosis
   B. Cluster headache
   C. Conjunctivitis
   D. Epilepsy
   E. Impending eclampsia
   F. Intracranial haemorrhage
   G. Malaria
   H. Meningitis
   I. Migraine
   J. Severe pre-eclampsia
   K. Sinusitis
   L. Subarachnoid haemorrhage
   M. Viral gastritis

1. A 27-year-old primigravid woman at 24 weeks of pregnancy is complaining of throbbing pain behind her left eye. This pain is so severe that she cannot sit still.

2. An 18-year-old primigravid woman at 36 weeks of pregnancy is complaining of sudden onset of headaches, abdominal pain, and a sensation of flashing lights in front of her eyes.

3. A 24-year-old multiparous woman at 30 weeks of pregnancy has returned from her holidays in Brazil. She is vomiting, feeling feverish, and complaining of severe headaches.

4. A 35-year-old parous woman at 20 weeks of pregnancy complains of severe headaches and feeling tired, feverish, and stiff around her neck.

5. A recently delivered multiparous woman with a BMI of 45 complains on day three post-partum of sudden onset of severe headache, describing it as the 'worst headache I ever had'.

Options for Questions 6–10

You have been called to see a collapsed patient. For each of the following clinical scenarios, choose the single most appropriate cause of collapse. Each option may be used once, more than once, or not at all.

   A. Diabetic ketoacidosis
   B. Hyperkalaemia
   C. Hypovolaemia
   D. Hypoxia
   E. Intracranial haemorrhage
   F. Myocardial infarction
   G. Sepsis
   H. Tamponade
   I. Tension pneumothorax
   J. Thromboembolism
   K. Toxicity

L. Concealed abruption

M. Vasovagal faint

6. You are asked to urgently see an unbooked pregnancy. She collapsed in A&E with constant severe abdominal pain. She has no vaginal bleeding. On examination she has a gravid uterus, approximately 34 cm, and you are unable to discern presentation due to a tense 'woody' abdomen. She smells heavily of cigarette smoke.

7. Your SHO calls you to A&E to see a woman day six following a normal vaginal delivery referred in by the GP. The referral letter tells you she had an induction at 38 weeks for severe pre-eclampsia, with no significant blood loss. She has had central chest pain for the last 12 hours.

8. You respond to the emergency buzzer call-out for room 6, a woman whom you delivered by ventouse four hours ago. She had a pudendal block. The blood loss was 400 ml and she had a oxytocin infusion. The midwife tells you that she stood up to go to the shower and fainted.

9. A woman attends triage four days after normal vaginal delivery of her fourth child. She had a first-degree tear which was not sutured. She gives a history of collapsing at home. She feels hot to the touch and looks pale. Her pulse rate is 120 bpm, with a blood pressure of 80/40. Her temperature is 37.4°C.

10. The ambulance brings in a 20-year-old unbooked woman who appears to be 27 weeks pregnant, following a collapse on the street. She is unkempt and smells of cigarette smoke. Examination is normal, with a soft, non-tender uterus. She is demanding pain relief but declines paracetamol. Her affect is somewhat confused and she hugs an agency midwife who recognizes her from a previous attendance at a different hospital.

Options for Questions 11–15

For each of the following clinical scenarios, choose the most appropriate course of management. Each option may be used once, more than once, or not at all.

A. Artificial rupture of membranes

B. Continuous external foetal monitoring

C. Encourage maternal effort

D. Commence pushing with consideration of an instrumental

E. Foetal scalp electrode

F. Grade 1 LSCS

G. Grade 2 LSCS

H. Intravenous access plus fluids

I. Kielland's forceps delivery

J. Neville Barnes forceps delivery

K. Reassess in two hours

L. Reassess in four hours

M. Rotational instrumental delivery

N. Stop oxytocin infusion

O. Syntocinon augmentation

P. Ventouse extraction

11. A 24-year-old primigravida undergoes IOL at 39/40 because of pre-eclampsia. Her BP was moderately raised on admission and her 24-hour protein was 3.5 g/24 hr. She was given prostaglandin and eight hours later is found to be 2 cm dilated. An ARM is performed with clear liquor draining. Oxytocinon infusion is commenced, and contractions are maintained at 4 in 10 minutes. Five hours later she is 7 cm dilated. After a further four hours, she is fully dilated. The presenting part is at the level of the ischial spines in LOA position, with 0/5th

palpable abdominally. There is some descent with maternal effort. Baseline rate is 140 bpm, variability 4 bpm; typical variable decelerations are present with most contractions for the past 50 minutes.

12. A 32-year-old primigravida is admitted in spontaneous labour at 34+ 6/40 gestation. Her cervix is 4 cm dilated. Epidural anaesthesia is administered at her request and continuous electronic foetal monitoring is commenced. Four hours later she is contracting 3 in 10, and there are typical variable decelerations with every contraction for the last 30 minutes. On examination she is fully dilated, the foetus presenting in direct occipito-anterior position, at level of ischial spines +1, with good descent on maternal effort. There is a loop of cord prolapsing beyond the foetal head.

13. A 35-year-old primigravida is admitted at 39/40 gestation, contracting 2 in 10 and found to be 3 cm dilated. She is HIV-positive with an undetectable viral load. Four hours later, she is found to be 4 cm dilated with no membranes felt. The presenting part is cephalic with 2/5th palpable per abdomen. CTG is normal.

14. A 35-year-old primigravida attends in spontaneous labour. She is found to be 3 cm dilated with absent membranes. An epidural is sited and continuous CTG monitoring commenced. She is contracting 4 in 10 minutes. Seven hours later she is found to be fully dilated, and passive descent is allowed. Two hours later the head is still at the level of the ischial spines, LOT. The baseline rate is 155 bpm, variability 6 bpm, no accelerations, and occasional typical variable decelerations with most contractions for the last ten minutes.

15. A 25-year-old multigravida is admitted to the labour ward at 28 weeks gestation with intermittent abdominal pain. The foetal heart is auscultated at 150 bpm with no decelerations noted. On examination there is mild uterine tenderness and the uterus is 30-weeks size. The cervix is fully dilated, with presentation extended breech, and heavily bloodstained liquor.

Options for Questions 16–20

For each of the following clinical scenarios, choose the most appropriate course of management on the ovarian cysts found in premenopausal women. Each option may be used once, more than once, or not at all.

A. AFP, HCG
B. AFP, LDH, HCG
C. CA125
D. CA125, AFP
E. CA125, AFP, LDH
F. CA125, AFP, LDH, HCG
G. CT scan
H. Discharge
I. Discuss with gynae-oncologist
J. Laparoscopy and aspiration of cyst
K. Laparoscopy and removal of cyst
L. Laparotomy
M. MRI
N. Prescribe COCP
O. Refer to gynae-oncologist
P. Repeat ultrasound
Q. Repeat USS in 3–6 months
R. Repeat USS in one year

16. A 34-year-old woman presents with an incidental finding of an ovarian cyst following an ultrasound for renal colic. The ultrasound shows a 30 mm thin smooth-walled unilocular cyst.

17. A 28-year-old woman is under investigation by the gynaecologists for chronic pelvic pain. Routine ultrasound shows a persistent thin-walled unilocular cyst (50 mm) with ground glass shadowing and echogenic foci.

18. A 36-year-old woman is seen in clinic with weight loss and abdominal pain. Ultrasound shows an irregular solid lesion close to the ovary with ascites and blood flow.

19. A 38-year-old woman presents with abdominal discomfort. Ultrasound shows bilateral hyperechoic masses (68 mm) with multiple thin echogenic lines and calcifications.

20. A 30-year-old woman presents with bleeding following a termination of pregnancy. Ultrasound is requested to look for retained products. No retained products of conception are found, but there is an area adjacent to the ovary with multiple thick septations and focal thickening of the lesion wall with a solid component.

Options for Questions 21–25

The following list of options contains approximate risk frequencies for complications associated with therapeutic abortion. For each complication described, choose the most appropriate risk frequency. Each option may be used once, more than once, or not at all.

    A. 1 in 10
    B. 5 in 100
    C. 2 in 100
    D. 1 in 100
    E. 4 in 1,000
    F. 2 in 1,000
    G. 3 in 1,000
    H. 1 in 1,000
    I. 1 in 10,000
    J. 1 in 12,500
    K. 1 in 15,000
    L. No increased risk

21. The risk of a failed first trimester medical or surgical induced abortion.

22. The risk of haemorrhage (blood loss > 500 ml) during first trimester medical or surgical abortion.

23. The risk of breast cancer following medical or surgical abortion.

24. The risk of uterine perforation at the time of first trimester surgical abortion.

25. Damage to the external cervical os at the time of surgical induced abortion.

Options for Questions 26–30

For each of the following clinical scenarios, choose the single most appropriate diagnosis. Each option may be used once, more than once, or not at all.

    A. Ectopic pregnancy
    B. Heterotopic pregnancy
    C. Inevitable miscarriage
    D. Missed miscarriage
    E. Molar pregnancy
    F. Ovarian pregnancy

G. Pregnancy of unknown location

H. Pregnancy of unknown viability

I. Retained products of conception

J. Threatened miscarriage

K. Twin pregnancy

L. Viable intrauterine pregnancy

26. A 23-year-old woman who is at six weeks gestation by dates is referred with vaginal spotting, which continues today. Examination shows a soft, non-tender abdomen and a closed cervical os. Ultrasound shows a CRL of 7 mm with foetal heart present. The ovaries and adnexa appear normal.

27. A 33-year-old primiparous woman is referred to the early pregnancy unit at approximately 12 weeks gestation with a history of vaginal spotting three days ago, which has now settled. Today she has no bleeding and is feeling well. Ultrasound shows a grape-like appearance to the endometrium. The ovaries and adnexa appear normal.

28. A 22-year-old woman who is at ten weeks gestation by dates is referred to the early pregnancy unit by the on-call gynae SHO for a scan. She was admitted with hyperemesis. She has no pain or vaginal bleeding. Ultrasound shows a foetal pole with a CRL of 8 mm. There is no foetal heart action noted. The ovaries and adnexa appear normal.

29. A 25-year-old woman who is at seven weeks gestation by dates self-refers to the early pregnancy unit due to a history of previous left ectopic pregnancy, treated with methotrexate. Ultrasound shows a gestational sac of 30 mm with a CRL of 6 mm. No foetal heart action is noted. The ovaries and adnexa appear normal.

30. A 33-year-old woman who is six weeks gestation by dates is referred by GP with a history of left-sided discomfort and feeling dizzy. BP is 120/70 and pulse 90 bpm. A transvaginal scan shows a thickened endometrium and an ill-defined mass in the left adnexa. There is a small amount of free fluid in the pouch of Douglas.

Options for Questions 31–35

For each of the following clinical scenarios, choose the single diagnosis most suitable from the list provided. Each option may be used once, more than once, or not at all.

A. Carcinoma of the bladder

B. Mixed urinary incontinence

C. Neurogenic bladder

D. Overactive bladder

E. Overflow incontinence

F. Painful bladder syndrome (PBS)

G. Urethral caruncle

H. Urethral diverticulum

I. Urethral prolapse

J. Urinary stress incontinence

K. Urinary tract infection

L. Urogenital atrophy

M. Vesico-vaginal fistula

31. A 59-year-old nulliparous woman presents with recurrent dysuria and frequency worsening over the past six months. She smokes 20 cigarettes per day. Repeated MSUs at her GP have never demonstrated infection. Urinalysis demonstrates + + haematuria. You have sent a repeat MSU for microscopy, culture, and sensitivity.

32. A 28-year-old woman presents ten days after an anterior colporrhaphy for cystocele. She complains of feeling constantly damp vaginally and is having to wear pads continuously.

33. A 62-year-old postmenopausal woman presents with an eight-month history of dysuria and vulval pain. On examination, a pink exophytic lesion is observed at the urethral meatus.

34. A 46-year-old woman who has had three previous vaginal deliveries presents with a two-year deteriorating history of leakage of urine on coughing, sneezing, and during exercise. On examination, a moderate cystocele and rectocele are observed.

35. A 58-year-old woman presents with a nine-month history of urinary frequency, urgency, and pelvic pain. Investigations including urodynamics have been normal.

Options for Questions 36–40

For each of the following clinical scenarios, choose the single most appropriate management option from the list provided. Each option may be used once, more than once, or not at all.

    A. Diagnostic laparoscopy
    B. Etoposide, methotrexate, actinomycin, paclitaxel
    C. Etoposide, methotrexate, dactinomycin, cyclophosphamide, and vincristine
    D. Evacuation of the uterus with mifepristone, misoprostol, and syntocinon
    E. Evacuation of the uterus with misoprostol
    F. Hysteroscopy
    G. Laparotomy
    H. Methotrexate
    I. Methotrexate, folic acid, and a single chemotherapy agent
    J. Refer to a tertiary hospital
    K. Refer to the local specialist centre
    L. Register with the regional centre and ask for advice
    M. Repeat evacuation of the uterus
    N. Repeat HCG 48 hours
    O. Repeat serum HCG
    P. Syntocinon infusion
    Q. Treat as normal
    R. Ultrasound scan

36. A 21-year-old woman attended the hospital at six weeks of amenorrhoea and a positive home pregnancy test. A likely miscarriage was diagnosed on ultrasound and she opted for surgical evacuation. Products of conception demonstrated partial hydatidiform mole.

37. The same 21-year-old woman re-attends hospital 15 weeks later with persistent vaginal bleeding. Her serum HCG has risen to 6,000 mIU/ml.

38. A 43-year-old multiparous woman is diagnosed with gestational neoplastic disease three months following a surgical termination. Her serum HCG is 10,000 mIU/ml. She has two small (1 cm) metastases in the lung.

39. A 24-year-old multiparous woman is diagnosed with gestational trophoblastic neoplasia (GTN) six months following a partial mole and has a single 6 cm metastasis in the liver.

40. A 21-year-old primiparous woman who has had a previous molar pregnancy is now pregnant one year later. Her pregnancy appears to be progressing well. How would you manage her following delivery?

Options for Questions 41–47

For each of the following clinical scenarios, choose the single most appropriate treatment. Each option may be used once, more than once, or not at all.

A. Anti-Müllerian hormone
B. Bromocriptine
C. Clomiphene
D. Endometrial ablation
E. FSH stimulation
F. Laparoscopic ovarian suspension
G. Laparoscopic tubal reconstructive surgery
H. LHRH agonist
I. Oocyte cryopreservation
J. Ovarian endometrioma excision
K. Ovarian endometrioma fenestration
L. Reassurance
M. Removal of polypi at hysteroscopy
N. Unilateral salpingectomy

41. A 35-year-old woman with primary infertility for 30 months has right-sided hydrosalpinx. She is now on the waiting list for IVF.

42. A 30-year-old woman with primary infertility of four years duration, diagnosed with bilateral ovarian endometriomas, each approximately 6 cm in diameter.

43. A 38-year-old woman with primary infertility of 36 months duration, waiting for IVF, has an ultrasound scan showing multiple endometrial polyps.

44. A 25-year-old multiparous woman who has undergone pelvic radiation.

45. A 22-year-old nulliparous woman with a BMI 16, diagnosed with hypogonadotrophic hypogonadism-related amenorrhoea, seeking infertility treatment.

46. A 30-year-old woman with confirmed ovulatory cycles with raised prolactin of 760 (normal <360 mIU/L). She does not complain of headaches or nipple discharge.

47. A 42-year-old woman with primary infertility of eight years duration had a failed stimulated IVF cycle. What investigation prior to her next IVF cycle should be performed?

Options for Questions 48–50

For each of the following clinical scenarios, choose the single most appropriate option. Each option may be used once, more than once, or not at all.

A. Bladder damage
B. Chronic constipation
C. Dehydration
D. Diabetic ketoacidosis
E. Fluid overload
F. Intraperitoneal haemorrhage
G. Ovarian pregnancy
H. Pelvic haematoma
I. Postoperative pelvic sepsis
J. Postoperative pneumonia
K. Pulmonary embolism

L. Torsion of the ovarian cyst

M. Tubal ectopic pregnancy

N. Ureteric injury

O. Uterine perforation and fluid overload

P. Vesico-vaginal fistula

48. A 40-year-old woman has a difficult abdominal hysterectomy and bilateral salpingo-oophorectomy for severe endometriosis. She was administered with oestradiol implant following hysterectomy. She comes for review appointment four weeks later and tells you that she is wearing pads and feels 'as if she has lost control of her bladder'.

49. A 45-year-old woman with a BMI of 40 had a laparoscopic-assisted hysterectomy for multiple uterine fibroids. She had a spinal block along with a general anaesthetic. Twelve hours later, her pelvic drain remains clear, her pulse is 110 bpm, pO_2 92, and she is feeling very uncomfortable, with a distended and tender abdomen.

50. A 35-year-old woman had an abdominal hysterectomy and bilateral salpingo-oophorectomy for severe pelvic inflammatory disease and menorrhagia. Twenty-four hours later, she complains of severe left flank pain which is not responsive to analgesics. Her urine output is satisfactory but pink in colour and blood pressure is stable. The fluid in her drain is pink sero-sanguinous, approximately 500 ml in total.

Single Best Answers

1. A. 50 mGy

The accepted background cumulative dose of ionizing radiation during pregnancy is 50 mGy (5 rad), with little evidence to suggest any change in risk of major malformations at this level.

Eastwood K, Mohan A. Imaging in pregnancy. *TOG* 2019;21(4):255–62.

2. D. 50%

Shortening and stenosis of the vaginal epithelium is common following radiotherapy, with dyspareunia reported by 55% of women after treatment for cervical carcinoma.

Hadwin R, Petts G, Olaitan A. Treatment related morbidity in gynaecological cancers. *TOG* 2010;12:79–86.

3. C. There is an increased risk of post-partum haemorrhage

Pregnancies after UAE are at higher risk of miscarriage compared to pregnancies post-laparoscopic myomectomy.

Homer H, Saidogan E. Pregnancy outcomes after uterine artery embolisation for fibroids. *TOG* 2012;11:4.

4. C. Significant trauma to the cervix

Serious risks of surgical evacuation of the uterus for early pregnancy loss include diagnosed uterine perforation in up to one in 1,000 women (uncommon) and significant trauma to the cervix, which is also uncommon. Frequent risks include vaginal bleeding lasting up to two weeks, the need for a repeat surgical procedure, and localized pelvic infection.

RCOG Consent Advice 10. Surgical Management of Miscarriage and Removal of Persistent Placental or Fetal Remains. January 2018.

5. C. FFP is stored at −30°C and needs to be defrosted thoroughly prior to administration

A prothrombin time and activated partial thromboplastin time ratio above 1.5 is associated with an increased risk of a clinical coagulopathy, which requires correction with FFP. FFP is derived from whole blood and contains clotting factors. It is stored at −30°C and needs to be defrosted thoroughly prior to administration. Cryoprecipitate contains more fibrinogen than FFP and is used to correct hypofibrinogenaemia. A unit of concentrated red cells increases the haemoglobin by 1 g/dl and the haematocrit by 3%.

RCOG Green-top Guideline 52. Prevention and management of post-partum haemorrhage; December 2016.

Stainsby D, et al. *Guidelines on the management of massive blood loss*. London: British Committee for Standards in Haematology; 2006.

6. C. Consider breastfeeding prior to taking lamotrigine

Women with epilepsy should be encouraged to breastfeed as most anti-epileptic drugs cross into the breast milk in only minimal amounts (3–5% of maternal levels). However, women taking lamotrigine should be advised to breastfeed prior to taking their medication to

minimize neonatal exposure as it crosses into breast milk in much larger doses (30–50%).

Nelson-Piercy C. *Obstetric medicine*, 6th ed. Boca Raton: CRC Press; 2021.

7. D. Increased risk of pre-eclampsia

Pulmonary TB which is diagnosed late in pregnancy increases the risk of pre-eclampsia, acute respiratory failure, and preterm labour. Extrapulmonary TB affects the mother's health but does not alter the course of the pregnancy, mode of delivery, or the rate of pre-eclampsia.

Mahendru A, Gajjar K, Eddy J. Diagnosis and management of tuberculosis in pregnancy. *TOG* 2011;12:163–71.

8. B. The IUCD is associated with heavier menstrual bleeding and intermenstrual spotting

The IUCD inhibits fertilization and implantation. Women can use the IUCD after a previous ectopic pregnancy and there is no association with tubal infertility. There is no indication to remove the IUCD in asymptomatic women with *Actinomyces*-like organisms. Side effects of the IUCD include heavier menstrual bleeding, intermenstrual spotting, and dysmenorrhoea.

Ritchie J, Phelan N, Briggs P. Intrauterine contraception. *TOG* 2021;23:187–95.

9. E. Progestogen

Cyproterone acetate is a strong progestogen which reduces plasma luteinizing hormone levels, thereby lowering testosterone and androstenedione levels. It also acts as an anti-androgen peripherally. Spironolactone is a diuretic which acts as an aldosterone antagonist to reduce hirsutism.

Swingler R, Awala A, Gordon U. Hirsutism in young women. *TOG* 2009;11:101–7.

10. B. Foetal thyroxine levels may be affected

Both carbimazole and propylthiouracil cause agranulocytosis and are equally effective in pregnancy. Treatment dose can be either reduced or stopped in the second and third trimesters. Antithyroid medication is ineffective in cases of hyperemesis gravidarum because there is no increase in thyroid activity.

Nelson-Piercy C. *Obstetric medicine*, 6th ed. Boca Raton: CRC Press; 2021.

11. D. Refer to a gynaecology oncologist

Both the patient's symptoms and ultrasound findings suggest a suspicious lesion warranting a referral to the gynaecology oncology team.

NICE Guideline 122. Ovarian cancer: recognition and initial management; 2011.

12. A. Congenital absence of the vas deferens

Azoospermia with normal hormone levels suggests an obstructive cause such as congenital absence of the vas deferens, vasectomy, and infection.

Karavolos S, Panagiotopoulou N, Alahwany H, Martins da Silva S. An update on the management of male infertility. *TOG* 2020;22:267–74.

13. **C.** Lupus anticoagulant

Standard investigations to determine the aetiology of recurrent miscarriage should include lupus anticoagulant and anticardiolipin antibodies as well as factor V Leiden and protein S deficiency. Pelvic ultrasound is not a blood investigation.

Chester MR, Tirlapur A, Jayaprakasan K. Current management of recurrent pregnancy loss. *TOG* 2022; 24:260–71.

14. **C.** Pre-eclampsia

An isolated high level of inhibin A in the second trimester is associated with preterm delivery, pre-eclampsia, low birthweight, and intrauterine death.

Lakhi N, Govind A, Moretti M, Jones J. Maternal serum analytes as markers of adverse obstetric outcome. *TOG* 2012;14:267–73.

15. **D.** A term baby admitted to the neonatal unit

The admission of a term baby to the neonatal unit should be investigated to identify any preventable factors. A stillbirth of 500 g should be reported. A baby born with Apgar scores below 7 at five minutes should be reported. An estimated blood loss over 1,500 ml at delivery should be reported. Successful vaginal breech deliveries do not trigger incident reports.

RCOG Clinical Governance Advice 2. Improving patient safety: risk management for maternity and gynaecology; 2009.

16. **A.** A 1 in 100 risk of bladder injury requiring repair

There is an increased risk of antepartum stillbirth: 1–4 in every 1,000 women. Risk of bladder damage is around 1 in 1,000 CS. The risk of foetal laceration at CS is 1–2 per 100 procedures. There is an increased risk of repeat emergency CS when vaginal delivery is attempted in subsequent pregnancies (one in every four women).

RCOG Consent Advice 7. Caesarean section; 2022.

17. **E.** Transected hymen

All are a variation of normal anatomy with the exception of a transected hymen. A hymenal transection is described as a (healed) discontinuity in the hymenal membrane that extends through the width of the hymen. This type of injury is thought to be strongly suggestive of a penetrative injury.

Wyatt J, Payne-James J, Norfolk G, Squires T. *Oxford handbook of forensic medicine*. Oxford: Oxford University Press; 2015.

18. **B.** Phenobarbitone crosses the placenta but carbamazepine does not

Valproate, phenobarbitone, carbamazepine, and primidone all cross the placenta. Phenytoin and valproate are associated with congenital heart defects. The risk of teratogenicity increases with the number of drugs. For patients taking two or more anticonvulsants the risk is 15%. For those taking valproate, carbamazepine, and phenytoin, the risk is as high as 50%. The teratogenic effect of valproate is dose-dependent. The risk of teratogenicity increases sixfold in mothers taking more than 1 g of valproate per day. Benzodiazepines including clonazepam are not teratogenic.

Nelson-Piercy C. *Obstetric medicine*, 6th ed. Boca Raton: CRC Press; 2021.

19. A. 250 IU

Surgical or medical management of ectopic pregnancy requires anti-D therapy.

Green-top Guideline 65. The management of women with red cell antibodies during pregnancy; 2014.

20. B. Capillary refill time

Cardiac output (CO), stroke volume (SV), and heart rate (HR) increase in pregnancy. Remember, CO = SV × HR. SV is the amount of blood pumped through the ventricles in one heartbeat. Therefore, CO is the amount of blood pumped through the ventricles in one minute. In pregnancy, CO increases by approximately 40%, from 4.5 L/minute to approximately 6 L/minute. This is due to a 30% increase in SV and 10% increase in HR. Blood volume increases by 30% in pregnancy. By comparison, plasma volume increases by 40%. This leads to a dilutional anaemia in pregnancy, which is most obvious in the first trimester.

Nelson-Piercy C. *Obstetric medicine*, 6th ed. Boca Raton: CRC Press; 2021.

21. B. Expulsion, occurring in 5% of cases

The risk of perforation with the intrauterine devices is uncommon, at less than 1 in 1,000. Expulsion of a device occurs in about 5% of women, usually in the first three months following insertion.

Ritchie, J, Phelan, N, Briggs, P. Intrauterine contraception. *TOG* 2021;23:187–95.

22. C. Refer to specialist unit for an ultrasound to measure the middle cerebral peak systolic velocity

All women who have anti-C antibody titres above 20 IU/ml should be referred to a specialist unit for investigation. To increase oxygen supply, the anaemic foetus increases its CO, which increases blood flow velocity. This is monitored by measuring the middle cerebral peak systolic velocity.

Castleman J, Gurney L, Kilby M, Morris RK. Identification and management of fetal anaemia: a practical guide. *TOG* 2021;23(3):196–205.

Gajjar K, Spencer C. Diagnosis and management of non-anti-D red cell antibodies in pregnancy. *TOG* 2009;11:89–95.

Green-top Guideline 65. The management of women with red cell antibodies during pregnancy; May 2014.

23. D. 14 days

The incubation period for rubella virus is 14–21 days. Women are infectious from seven days before and until seven days after the onset of the rash.

To M, Kidd M, Maxwell D. Prenatal diagnosis and management of fetal infections. *TOG* 2009;11(2):108–16.

24. E. Prescribe thromboprophylaxis

The management of OHSS is dictated by its severity. Analgesia should be prescribed for pain, with strict fluid balance. An ascitic tap should be considered if the patient is clinically short of breath or in constant significant abdominal pain. Antibiotics should be considered only where infection is suspected.

Prakash A, Mathur R. Ovarian hyperstimulation syndrome. *TOG* 2013;15:31–5.

25. B. *BRCA* mutation carriers have a better prognosis for ovarian cancer than non-carriers

The estimated risk of ovarian cancer is 35–40% for *BRCA1* mutation carriers and 13–23% for *BRCA2* mutation carriers. *BRCA* carriers are more likely to have invasive serous adenocarcinoma, but the stage of presentation is similar to that of the general population. Ovarian cancers in *BRCA* mutation carriers are more likely to be of higher grade than ovarian cancers in age-matched controls. *BRCA* mutation carriers, especially BRCA2 carriers, have a better prognosis than non-carriers.

Gaughan E, Walsh T. Risk-reducing surgery for women at high risk of epithelial ovarian cancer. *TOG* 2014;16:185–91..

26. C. Placental chorioangioma

Maternal causes of polyhydramnios include uncontrolled diabetes mellitus, Rhesus, and other blood group isoimmunization, and exposure to medications such as lithium, which leads to foetal diabetes insipidus. Foetal causes include anencephaly, spina bifida, hydrocephalus, foetal goitre, cystic hygroma, cleft palate, exomphalos, gastroschisis, and cardiac anomalies. Placental causes include tumours such as chorioangiomas.

Karkhanis P, Patni S. Polyhydramnios in singleton pregnancies; perinatal outcomes and management. *TOG* 2014;16:207–13.

27. A. A blood loss of over 40% of total blood volume of a 70-kg woman is considered 'life-threatening'

Allowing for the physiological increase in pregnancy, total blood volume at term is approximately 100 ml/kg (an average 70-kg woman will have a total blood volume of 7,000 ml). A blood loss of more than 40% of total blood volume (approximately 2,800 ml) is generally regarded as 'life-threatening'. Prophylactic oxytocics given routinely in the management of the third stage of labour in all women reduce the risk of PPH by only about 60%. It is common practice to administer oxytocin (5 IU by slow intravenous injection) during CS to encourage uterine contraction. However, there are scenarios where a low-dose infusion would be more appropriate (e.g. in women with severe cardiovascular conditions). Ergometrine is contraindicated for prophylaxis in women known to be hypertensive, but in severe PPH where the uterus has not responded to other uterotonic drugs, ergometrine may still be used. Misoprostol is not as effective as oxytocin in the management of PPH.

RCOG Green-top Guideline No. 27a. Placenta praevia and placenta accreta: diagnosis and management; 2018.

RCOG Green-top Guideline 47. Blood transfusion in obstetrics; 2015.

RCOG Green-top Guideline 52. Prevention and management of postpartum haemorrhage; 2016.

28. E. There is a risk of significant regret

Selective foetal reduction leads to a decrease in foetal mortality and short- and long-term morbidity of the remaining twin. There is a 10% risk of miscarriage. Selective foetal reduction is associated with a significant amount of guilt or regret.

RCOG Evidence-based Clinical Guideline Number 7. The Care of Women Requesting Induced Abortion; 2011.

29. E. The use of FISH reduces the delay in obtaining a result for amniocentesis

Amniocentesis is usually performed at 15–16 weeks gestation. The main disadvantages are the 0.5% culture failure, the 0.5–1% increased miscarriage rate, and the delay in obtaining a result (although this is reduced by using FISH). CVS is performed from 11 weeks gestation. A result is obtained more swiftly than with amniocentesis, but the miscarriage rate is up to 2%.

RCOG Green-top Guideline 8. Amniocentesis and chorionic villus sampling; 2021.

30. D. Progestogens can be used to treat metropathia haemorrhagica

Progestogens can be used to treat anovulatory dysfunctional bleeding, particularly metropathia haemorrhagica. To stop an acute episode, continuous progestogen can be used for up to 21 days. In ovulatory menorrhagia, antifibrinolytics and NSAIDs are more effective. There is no evidence that progestogens are useful in treating PMS.

NICE Guideline 44. Heavy menstrual bleeding: assessment and management; 2018.

31. D. Thalassaemia major is associated with cardiac failure

She may have a degree of anaemia requiring folate supplementation and oral iron if iron-deficient. Parenteral iron is contraindicated because of the risk of hepatic damage. Given her fiancé is of the same ethnic background, there is an increased risk of haemoglobinopathy, so pre-pregnancy screening should be offered. If her fiancé is screened positive, there is a 25% chance that the baby will suffer from beta thalassaemia major. Thalassaemia major is associated with liver dysfunction, diabetes, and cardiac failure, which can lead to death.

RCOG Green-top Guideline 66. Management of beta thalassaemia in pregnancy; 2014.

32. E. Transverse presentation

Risk factors for umbilical cord prolapse include multiparity, prematurity, uterine malformations, malpresentations, instrumental delivery, and ARM.

RCOG Green-top Guideline 50. Umbilical cord prolapse; 2014.

33. E. Tumour size

Women with a FIGO score ≤6 are at low risk and receive single-agent chemotherapy with methotrexate. If their score is ≥6 they require multiagent chemotherapy. Age, not parity, is a criterion. Mole, abortion, or term pregnancy results in scores of 0, 1, and 2, respectively. Tumour size, including the uterus (in cm), is a criterion. Lung, spleen and kidney, gut, liver, and brain sites of metastases form part of the scoring system. Other criteria include interval months from the end of antecedent pregnancy to treatment, pretreatment serum HCG (IU/L), and number of metastases.

RCOG Green-top Guideline 39. The management of gestational trophoblastic disease; 2020.

34. E. 70%

The risk of vertical transmission of parvovirus B19 is 15% in women under 15 weeks gestation, 25% between 15 and 20 weeks, rising to 70% at term.

To M, Kidd M, Maxwell D. Prenatal diagnosis and management of fetal infections. *TOG* 2009;11:108–16.

35. C. 330

RMI = U×M×CA125. U, ultrasound scan, is scored 1 point for a multilocular cyst, evidence of solid areas, metastases, ascites, or bilateral lesions. M = 3 for all postmenopausal women. Here, ultrasound score is 2 (multilocular and solid areas); therefore RMI = 2×3×55.

RCOG Green-top Guideline 34. Ovarian cysts in post-menopausal women; 2016.

36. E. Recurrence rate is affected by maternal age

Almost 95% of cases are due to meiotic non-disjunction, 2% result from Robertsonian translocation, 2% result from mosaicism, and 1% are due to chromosomal rearrangements.

About 40–50% of babies with Down's will have congenital heart problems such as VSD, PDA, and AVSD. The risk of recurrence is influenced by maternal age and parental germline mosaicism. If the father carries a Robertsonian translocation, the risk of recurrence is <1%; if the mother carries it, the recurrence rate is 10–15%. After two affected foetuses the recurrence rate is approximately 10%.

Kumar S. *Handbook of fetal medicine*. Cambridge: Cambridge University Press; 2010, pp. 3–4.

37. D. Reassure and discharge to GP

This woman's presenting symptom is unrelated to the finding of a polyp. She does not complain of abnormal bleeding; given her age, conservative management is indicated.

Annan J, et al. The management of endometrial polyps in the 21st century. *TOG* 2012;14(1):33–8.

Wang JH, et al. Opportunities and risk factors for premalignant and malignant transformation of endometrial polyps: management strategies. *J Minim Invasive Gynecol* 2010;17:53–8.

38. C. Previously unsuccessful incontinence surgery

Videourodynamics also yields information about the anatomy of the urinary tract which is useful where there has been previous surgery (to assess bladder neck elevation), neuropathic bladder (bladder diverticula and trabeculation may be visualized), or anatomical defects (e.g. ectopic ureter).

NICE Clinical Guideline 123. Urinary incontinence and pelvic organ prolapse in women: management; 2019.

39. D. Colostrum is produced in small quantities after the birth of the baby

Colostrum does not have high levels of carbohydrate. Colostrum is produced in small quantities after the birth of the baby. Breastfeeding should be initiated within one hour of birth to maximize success. In the UK, about a fifth of mothers are still breastfeeding at six months. Colostrum is especially rich in IgA.

Collins S, Arulkumaran S, Hayes K, Jackson S, Impey L, eds. *Oxford handbook of obstetrics and gynaecology*. Oxford: Oxford University Press; 2013, chap. 9.

40. E. Pulsatile gonadotrophin-releasing hormone

In hypothalamic hypogonadism, changes in lifestyle to achieve a healthy BMI and pulsatile administration of gonadotrophin-releasing hormone or gonadotrophins with luteinizing hormone is the therapy for ovulation induction, not clomiphene.

NICE Clinical Guideline 156. Fertility problems: assessment and treatment; 2013.

41. A. More than 90% of the UK antenatal population are seropositive for varicella zoster IgG

As the varicella vaccine is live, it is advised that the vaccine is not given in pregnancy, and that pregnancy is avoided for three months following vaccination. Varicella pneumonia occurs in up to 10% of cases in pregnancy and can be fatal. Severity worsens with increasing gestation. Varicella pneumonia occurs in up to 10% of cases in pregnancy and can be fatal. Severity worsens with increasing gestation. Chickenpox does not increase the risk of spontaneous miscarriage in the first trimester. However, infection at this stage means that the foetus is at risk of foetal varicella syndrome.

RCOG Green-top Guideline 13. Chickenpox in pregnancy; 2015.

42. D. Prescribe intravenous antihypertensive treatment

This qualifies as severe hypertension. The priority here therefore is to treat the blood pressure.

NICE Clinical Guideline 107. Hypertension in pregnancy: diagnosis and management; 2010.

43. C. Migraine

A migraine is classically pulsating, unilateral, moderate-to-severe in intensity, associated with nausea, vomiting, sensitivity to light and sound, and lasts hours. It is aggravated by routine physical activity.

Revell K, Morrish P. Headaches in pregnancy. *TOG* 2014;16:179–84.

44. A. Genital piercing

Type 1 FGM refers to the partial or total removal of the clitoris and prepuce; type 2 refers to partial or total removal of the clitoris and labia minora. Type 3 refers to infibulation (narrowing of the vaginal orifice by creating a covering seal by cutting and appositioning the labia minora), and type 4 refers to all other harmful procedures to the female genitalia. This includes genital piercing, cauterization, pricking, and incising.

RCOG Green-top Guideline 53. Female genital mutilation and its management; July 2015.

45. D. Protection from Alzheimer's disease

Postmenopausal HRT reduces bone loss, oestrogenizes the lower genital tract, and reduces the risk of colonic cancer (just like combined oral contraceptive pill). It does increase risk of VTE. Therefore risk identification is important before starting HRT. Data are conflicting regarding HRT's role in preventing Alzheimer's disease.

NICE Guideline 23. Menopause: diagnosis and management; 2015

Santen RJ, et al. Postmenopausal hormone therapy: an Endocrine Society scientific statement. *J Clin Endocrinol Metab* 2010;95(Suppl 1):S1–S66.

46. E. Struma ovarii

This is a type of dermoid cyst with active thyroid tissue. In almost 10% of women, enough thyroxine is produced to cause hyperthyroidism.

NICE Guideline 122. Ovarian cancer: recognition and initial management; 2011.

47. C. Posterior vaginal wall repair

The diagnosis here is posterior vaginal wall prolapse. The risk factors include multiparity and chronic constipation. Whilst pelvic floor exercises are effective at strengthening pelvic floor musculature, the definitive management of stage 2–3 vaginal wall prolapse is surgical.

NICE Guideline 171. Urinary incontinence in women: management; 2013.

48. D. Metoclopramide

Physiological causes include pregnancy, breastfeeding, and stress. Pathological causes of hyperprolactinaemia include prolactinomas, chronic renal failure, hypothyroidism, lung cancer, and sarcoidosis. Women with PCOS may have mildly elevated prolactin levels. Alpha-methyldopa is a dopamine agonist, which therefore stimulates prolactin production. Metoclopramide is a dopamine agonist which can cause hyperprolactinaemia.

Luesley, DM, Baker PN, eds. *Obstetrics and gynaecology: an evidence-based text for MRCOG*, 2nd ed. Boca Raton: CRC Press; 2010.

49. C. Granulosa cell tumours

Granulosa theca cell tumours from the ovaries produce oestrogen, which does not respond to hypothalamic feedback, thus leading to high circulating levels of oestrogen. This unopposed oestrogen can stimulate the endometrium and lead to endometrial cancer.

RCOG Scientific Impact Paper No. 52. Management of female malignant ovarian germ cell tumours; November 2016

50. A. Antimuscarinic

Oxybutynin is one of several drugs recommended in the treatment of overactive bladder.

NICE Guideline 171. Urinary incontinence in women: management; 2013.

Extended Matching Questions

Answers for Questions 1–5

1. B; 2. E; 3. G; 4. H; 5. A

1. Cluster headaches are uncommon and affect men more often than women. The word 'cluster' is used as the sufferers get a number of attacks over a few weeks and thereafter they are symptom-free for months or years. Cluster headaches normally present with severe headache which is much worse than migraine. The pain usually occurs at the same time each day and quite often wakens the individual a few hours after they have gone to sleep. Migraine is usually categorized according to whether or not there is aura.

2. Impending eclampsia, as this patient has risk factors such as being primigravida, under 20, and has sudden onset of headache and flashing lights. Her abdominal pain may be suggestive of perihepatic capsular congestion.

3. A history of travel is reported; therefore the most likely diagnosis is cerebral malaria, which is suggestive of severe headache and vomiting.

4. Meningitis is highly likely; the only giveaway would be that petechial rash has not been mentioned, which could be suggestive of meningococcal infection.

5. Cerebrovascular thrombosis usually occurs post-partum and has been noted even in the first trimester in the confidential enquiries into maternal deaths. Patients usually describe it as 'the worst I ever had' headache. In the presence of leucocytosis, differential diagnosis will include puerperal sepsis.

MBRRACE-UK Saving Lives, Improving Mothers' Care—Lessons learned to inform maternity care from the UK and Ireland Confidential Enquiries into Maternal Deaths and Morbidity 2017-19; 2021.

Answers for questions 6–10

6. L; 7. J; 8. M; 9. G; 10. K

6. Concealed abruption is the most likely cause of the abdominal pain and collapse.

7. This woman is at high risk for VTE, with a history suggesting a PE.

8. The history here is suggestive of a vasovagal faint, but you must always look for evidence of PPH as she has a prolonged second stage.

9. The most likely cause here is severe sepsis causing hypotension and hypovolemia.

10. The scenario suggests toxicity as the likely explanation of this presentation, possibly with alcohol or other drugs. A full neurological examination is indicated, along with a full social services workup.

RCOG Green-top Guideline 64a. Bacterial sepsis in pregnancy; 2012

Answers for questions 11–15

11. D; 12. J; 13. O; 14. C; 15. B

11. As the CTG is pathological (reduced variability and decelerations are present), either a foetal blood sample or delivery should be considered the most appropriate management. Here, a foetal blood sample would be optimal first-line management, given this woman's progress.

12. In keeping with RCOG Green-top Guidelines, Neville Barnes forceps delivery can be considered in women who are fully dilated with cord prolapse.

13. Here, syntocinon augmentation should be considered given the contraction frequency is suboptimal at 2 in 10.

14. Following two hours of passive descent, women should be encouraged to push actively for one hour.

15. Continuous monitoring is essential to monitor foetal well-being; in a multiparous woman, a preterm breech delivery is likely, but the risk associated with the aftercoming head should be considered.

NICE Clinical Guideline 190. Intrapartum care for healthy women and babies; 2014

Answers for questions 16–20

16. H; 17. K; 18. O; 19. Q; 20. B

16. The scan shows a simple asymptomatic cyst.

17. This describes a persistent endometrioma. The question indicates that there have been repeated ultrasound scans and therefore it is best to proceed to a laparoscopic removal.

18. IOTA M rules. This describes a suspicious lesion and needs immediate referral to the gynaecology oncology team.

19. This requires a repeat ultrasound scan in 3–6 months and follow-up. Should it be persistent, a laparoscopy may be indicated.

20. This describes a suspicious lesion, which may be a germ cell considering the history.

RCOG/BSGE Joint Green-top Guideline 62. Management of suspected ovarian masses in premenopausal women; 2011.

Answers for Questions 21–25

21. D; 22. H; 23. L; 24. E; 25. D

These are the risks as stated in the reference below. The risk of uterine perforation is moderate at 1–4 in 1,000; risk of haemorrhage is 1 in 1,000 overall; risk of cervical trauma is moderate at 1 in 100; risk of first trimester abortion failure is 2.3 in 1,000 (surgical) and 1–14 in 1,000 (medical). Induced abortion is not associated with an increase in breast cancer risk.

RCOG Evidence-based Clinical Guideline 7. The care of women requesting induced abortion; November 2011.

Answers for Questions 26–30

26. J; 27. E; 28. D; 29. H; 30. A

26. This patient has a viable intrauterine pregnancy; however, the continued spotting suggests this is better classified as a threatened miscarriage.

27. The grape-like appearance is typical of ultrasound scan findings for a molar pregnancy.

28. There is an empty sac at seven weeks of gestation; therefore a diagnosis of missed miscarriage should be considered.

29. Although the gestational sac is greater than 25 mm, there is an embryo seen, and if an embryo is seen, its measurements are used to aid diagnosis. Therefore, with a CRL <7 mm, no foetal heart is expected. Therefore this is a pregnancy of unknown viability.

30. This is a case of an ectopic pregnancy, as noted by her symptoms and signs. Her ultrasound scan shows blood in the pouch of Douglas which explains her dizziness. Ovarian ectopic pregnancy is very rare.

NICE Guideline 126. Ectopic pregnancy and miscarriage: diagnosis and initial management; 2019.

RCOG Green-top Guideline 21. Diagnosis and management of ectopic pregnancy; 2016.

Answers for Questions 31–35

31. A; 32. M; 33. G; 34. J; 35. F

31. Carcinoma in situ of the bladder can present with urinary symptoms. Haematuria should always be investigated before treating urinary symptoms as benign. Cystoscopy and cytology are other investigations that could be performed.

32. Unrecognized bladder injury during vaginal repair may lead to the development of a vesico-vaginal fistula. Incontinence is unlikely to leave a person constantly damp, especially at this woman's age.

33. Urethral caruncles are benign, distal urethral lesions that are most commonly found in postmenopausal women. Urethral prolapse is similar in appearance, but is circumferential, while caruncles are focal. Urethral prolapse may occur in prepubescent or postmenopausal females, whereas caruncles are seen almost exclusively in the latter.

34. Urinary stress incontinence most often presents in parous women and classically deteriorates over time.

35. PBS is defined as an unpleasant sensation (pain, pressure, discomfort) perceived to be related to the urinary bladder and associated with lower urinary tract symptoms of more than six weeks duration, in the absence of infection or other identifiable causes.

NICE Guideline 171. Urinary incontinence in women: management; 2013.

Answers for Questions 36–40

36. K; 37. R; 38. I; 39. C; 40. L

36. All women diagnosed with molar pregnancy should be referred for follow-up at the regional GTD centre. No further intervention is required immediately after the diagnosis if the uterus was evacuated. Her histology will be reviewed to confirm the diagnosis. If this is confirmed, she requires monitoring with serial HCG measurements only.

37. An ultrasound scan is the first investigation to determine if this is a second pregnancy or if there is persistent GTD. If GTN is diagnosed, then referral for chemotherapy treatment is required but it is essential to exclude a normal intrauterine pregnancy first.

38. See Table 1.1 for the FIGO scoring system. A score of less than 6 requires single-agent chemotherapy with methotrexate and folic acid.

Table 1.1 FIGO staging for gestational trophoblastic neoplasia (GTN) 2000

FIGO score	0	1	2	4
Age	<40	>40	–	–
Previous pregnancy	Mole	Abortion	Term	–
Interval months from end of index pregnancy to treatment	<4	4–7	7–13	>13
Pretreatment serum HCG	<1,000	1,000–10,000	10,000–100,000	>100,000
Largest tumour size	<3 cm	3–5 cm	>5 cm	–
Metastatic site	Lung	Spleen, kidney	Gut	Liver, brain
Number of metastases	–	1–4	5–8	>8
Previous failed chemotherapy	–	–	Single drug	Two or more drugs

Adapted from *International Journal of Gynecology & Obstetrics*, 77.3, FIGO Oncology Committee, 'FIGO staging for gestational trophoblastic neoplasia 2000 FIGO Oncology Committee', pp. 285–7, Copyright (2002), with permission from Elsevier and FIGO International Federation of Gynecology and Obstetrics.

39. Despite the lack of clinical information provided here, it can be calculated that her score is more than 6 and she therefore requires multiagent chemotherapy.

40. This patient should be registered with one of the hydatidiform mole centres. Watch for signs of pregnancy complications, such as PET. Discuss arrangements for follow-up post-delivery. Such patents require HCG follow-up post-delivery.

RCOG Green-top Guideline 38. The management of gestational trophoblastic disease; 2020.

Answers for Questions 41–47

41. N; 42. J; 43. M; 44. F; 45. E; 46. L; 47. A

41. The presence of a hydrosalpinx reduces implantation rate, therefore a salpingectomy or clipping of the affected tube should be considered prior to assisted conception treatment.

42. Ovarian endometrioma excision should be considered as endometriomas reduce ovarian reserve. There is evidence that prior surgery for ovarian endometriomas of >3 cm can improve pregnancy rates.

43. The most recent randomized studies have suggested that visible polypi should be removed at hysteroscopy before offering IVF treatment.

44. Laparoscopic ovarian suspension should be considered for women who are going for pelvic radiation treatment. An alternative option would be to undertake ovarian biopsy and cryopreserve tissue which can be used later for re-implantation of ovarian tissue in the ovarian cortex.

45. This is a case of hypogonadotrophic hypogonadism amenorrhea and should be treated with gonadotrophic stimulation.

46. Reassurance is key as this woman has had confirmed ovulatory cycles with raised prolactin below 1,000. If she is asymptomatic no treatment with bromocriptine is indicated.

47. Estimation of anti-Müllerian hormone (AMH) is a good predictor of response to IVF stimulation, especially among those who are above 40 and where fertility potential is already low.

Hung E, Ng Y, Ho PC. Subfertility: current concepts in management. *Best Pract Res Clin Obstet Gynaecol* 2012;26(6).

Answers for Questions 48–50

48. P; 49. F; 50. N

48. Difficult surgery for severe pelvic endometriosis is a clue to either damage to the bladder, where uterovesicular reflection is dissected (vesico-vaginal fistula) or damage to one of the ureters, which has been crushed or dissected. Some patients may even present with symptoms of detrusor instability.

49. Drains quite often get blocked, therefore full assessment of the patient is indicated. Here, significant intraperitoneal bleeding has caused her discomfort and tachycardia.

50. Difficult surgery is always a risk factor for ureteric injury/ligation. If the ureter has been transected, then hydroureter and hydronephrosis develop which gives constant flank pain.

Guideline of European Society of Human Reproduction and Embryology. Endometriosis; 2022.

Single Best Answers

1. **You are pre-assessing a 49-year-old woman who is due to undergo a radical hysterectomy for endometrial carcinoma. On discussing the risk of fistulae formation, she asks you when this is likely to present clinically.**
   A. Within 24 hours of the operation
   B. Within 48 hours of the operation
   C. Within the first five days postoperatively
   D. Between five and fourteen days postoperatively
   E. After four weeks postoperatively

2. **You review the blood results of a 26-year-old woman being investigated for recurrent pregnancy loss. The results show a haemolytic anaemia, low C4 level, and neutrophils of 2×10^9/L. What is the most likely diagnosis?**
   A. Acute myeloid leukaemia
   B. Antiphospholipid syndrome
   C. HIV
   D. Immune thrombotic thrombocytopaenia
   E. Systemic lupus erythematosus

3. **You review a 17-year-old woman who requests emergency contraception after four episodes of unprotected sexual intercourse over the last five days. She is asthmatic, with an admission to ITU last year. Which method of contraception is the most appropriate to prescribe?**
   A. Copper intrauterine device
   B. Levonorgestrel pill
   C. Mirena coil
   D. Progesterone-only pill
   E. Ulipristal acetate

4. **A 34-year-old woman is being consented for a caesarean section for placenta praevia. She has had a previous caesarean section. What is her chance of emergency hysterectomy?**
    A. Up to 11 in 1,000 women
    B. Up to 27 in 1,000 women
    C. Up to 7 in 100 women
    D. Up to 11 in 100 women
    E. Up to 27 in 100 women

5. **A 40-year-old woman who has a 20-pack-a-year history of smoking and a BMI of 35 presents with menorrhagia and dysmenorrhoea. What is the most appropriate form of medical management?**
    A. Aspirin
    B. Combined oral contraceptive pill
    C. Gonadotrophin-releasing hormone analogues
    D. Ibuprofen
    E. Mirena intrauterine system

6. **You are preparing a presentation on malignancy in pregnancy. What is the most common malignancy associated with pregnancy?**
    A. Bowel cancer
    B. Breast cancer
    C. Cervical cancer
    D. Ovarian cancer
    E. Thyroid cancer

7. **A 22-year-old woman presents with new-onset hirsutism. Her BMI is 19 and a pelvic ultrasound is normal. You note her testosterone level is 3 ng/ml, and her dehydroepiandrosterone sulphate level is also high. What is your diagnosis?**
    A. Acromegaly
    B. Adrenal tumour
    C. Cushing syndrome
    D. Ovarian Sertoli cell tumour
    E. Prolactinoma

8. **A 37-year-old woman presents at 13 weeks gestation, concerned about the risk of trisomy 21. She is keen to pursue an amniocentesis as soon as possible as she has been told it is more accurate than chorionic villus sampling. Which of the following is a risk if amniocentesis is done before 14 weeks of gestation?**
    A. Foetal talipes
    B. Increased risk of preterm labour
    C. Intrauterine growth restriction
    D. Oligohydramnios
    E. Placental mosaicism

9. You review a 23-year-old woman with cystic fibrosis for pre-conceptual counselling. Which of the following is correct regarding pregnancy in women with cystic fibrosis?

    A. The average life expectancy of women with cystic fibrosis in the UK is 55 years
    B. Fertility is reduced by approximately 30%
    C. The risk of miscarriage is unchanged when compared to the general population
    D. There is a higher incidence of congenital malformations
    E. There is an association with foetal growth restriction

10. You are called by the midwife to review a woman who presents with constant lower abdominal pain and fresh bleeding at 35 + 5 weeks gestation in her second pregnancy. Which of the following risk factors is most predictive of placental abruption?

    A. Advanced maternal age
    B. Obesity
    C. Pre-eclampsia
    D. Previous history of placental abruption
    E. Smoking

11. A 16-year-old girl is referred to your clinic with primary amenorrhoea. She is fit and well and has normal secondary sexual characteristics on examination. She is 170 cm tall and weighs 62 kg. Blood investigations and ultrasound are normal. What is the most likely diagnosis?

    A. Kallmann's syndrome
    B. Physiological causes
    C. Resistant ovary syndrome
    D. Turner's syndrome
    E. Uterovaginal agenesis

12. Whilst performing your antenatal morning ward round, you come across a 22-year-old woman in her first pregnancy at 37 weeks gestation who has been admitted with sickle cell crisis. She describes severe pain in her right arm, which is persistent. Which of the following is the most appropriate first-line management?

    A. Book the patient for an induction of labour as soon as possible
    B. Intramuscular pethidine
    C. Intravenous antibiotics
    D. Prescribe a blood transfusion
    E. Prescribe thromboprophylaxis

13. **You have been asked by your consultant to review the governance and standards of ultrasound training in your department. Which of the following would you undertake?**

    A. Develop an equipment replacement programme
    B. Ensure all ultrasound images are archived
    C. Review the evidence of training and continuing professional development in the department
    D. Review the maintenance and calibration checks for each ultrasound machine
    E. Review the reports of all examinations

14. **A 28-year-old pregnant woman is diagnosed with stage 2 breast cancer. Which of the following is true regarding management?**

    A. Reconstruction can be performed at the same time as surgical treatment
    B. Sentinel node assessment using radioisotope scintigraphy can be performed in pregnancy
    C. Surgical treatment can be undertaken from the second trimester onwards
    D. Systemic chemotherapy is contraindicated in the second trimester
    E. Trastuzumab should be given during pregnancy instead of tamoxifen

15. **A 24-year-old woman at 25 weeks gestation presents for advice following exposure to a child one week ago who developed chickenpox two days ago. Which of the following is true regarding the varicella-zoster virus (VZV)?**

    A. Following primary infection, the virus may not always remain dormant in the sensory nerve root ganglia
    B. HIV-positive women who develop chickenpox in pregnancy should be referred to hospital
    C. It is infectious 48 hours after the rash appears until the vesicles crust over
    D. VZIG should be given once a rash appears and chickenpox is diagnosed
    E. VZV is an RNA virus which is transmitted by respiratory droplets and direct personal contact

16. **A 22-year-old woman is diagnosed with polycystic ovary syndrome. She asks about the risks of cardiovascular disease, as her mother has recently been diagnosed with hypertension. Which one of the following is a true cardiovascular risk from PCOS?**

    A. An abnormal lipid profile mainly consists of raised high-density lipoprotein cholesterol
    B. Blood pressure ≥140/90 mmHg not responding to healthy lifestyle changes warrants drug therapy
    C. There is no need to rule out androgen-secreting tumours or serum 17-hydroxyprogesterone in cases with clinical evidence of hyperandrogenism
    D. Women with PCOS have a high prevalence of impaired glucose tolerance test and type 2 diabetes mellitus compared to the general population
    E. Women with PCOS have similar cardiovascular risks as weight-matched controls with normal ovarian function

17. **A 30-year-old woman presents with a worsening cough, night sweats, and feeling unwell at 24 weeks gestation. She is found to be sputum positive for Gram-positive, acid-fast bacilli, and a chest X-ray shows patch shadows in the upper zones with some fibrosis and areas of cavitation. Which of the following medications should be considered for treatment?**
    A. Amoxicillin and metronidazole
    B. Azithromycin and erythromycin
    C. Co-amoxiclav
    D. Isoniazid and rifampicin
    E. Zidovudine

18. **One of your patients requires a hysteroscopy for investigation of postmenopausal bleeding. Which one of the following is true regarding outpatient hysteroscopy?**
    A. It is contraindicated in women with a BMI greater than 40 kg/m²
    B. It may be achieved via the vaginoscopic route
    C. Menstruation prevents the procedure
    D. Operative procedures such as polypectomy will need to be performed under general anaesthetic
    E. This procedure is contraindicated in nulliparous women

19. **A 25-year-old woman presents in her second pregnancy at eight weeks gestation. She has previously had a painless preterm delivery at 26 weeks gestation, with no cause found. Which of the following is correct?**
    A. Cerclage is recommended for funnelling of the cervix without cervical shortening
    B. The insertion of a cerclage should be considered in women who have an incidentally identified short cervix of 25 mm length or less, regardless of their parity
    C. PPROM is not a contraindication to cervical cerclage
    D. Prophylactic cervical cerclage is recommended in women with a history of previous cervical cone biopsy
    E. Transabdominal cerclage can be performed in early pregnancy

20. **A 57-year-old woman consults you for a review of her HRT, which she has been taking for three years now. Which of the following is correct?**
    A. Bisphosphonates are used as primary prophylactic treatment to prevent fractures
    B. Clonidine can be used to treat vaginal dryness
    C. Combined HRT should not be given to women who have had a bilateral salpingo-oophorectomy for *BRCA* mutation
    D. Osteoporosis is confirmed with a T score of −2.5 on DEXA scan
    E. Prophylactic removal of the uterus is not essential in treating women who are carriers for Lynch syndrome

21. **A 28-year-old woman books late in pregnancy at approximately 28 weeks gestation. She is known to be hyperthyroid prior to pregnancy, but has stopped taking her medication due to the pregnancy. What risk is associated with uncontrolled hyperthyroidism?**
    A. Antepartum haemorrhage
    B. Diabetes
    C. Microcephaly
    D. Neonatal hyperthyroidism
    E. Polyhydramios

22. **You are asked to review a 56-year-old woman found to have a unilateral complex 7 cm ovarian cyst with some ascites. She is asymptomatic, and you calculate her RMI to be 265. Which of the following is correct management?**
    A. Perform a laparoscopic cystectomy
    B. Perform ultrasound-guided cyst aspiration
    C. Repeat ultrasound in four months
    D. Request an MRI and refer to gynaecology oncologist
    E. Request LDH

23. **You review a 34-year-old woman with pyrexia 48 hours following an emergency caesarean section. Which of the following antibiotics is correctly matched to its corresponding infection?**
    A. Clindamycin does not cover for anaerobic bacteria
    B. Co-amoxiclav is effective in treating methicillin-resistant *Staphylococcus aureus* (MRSA)
    C. Gentamicin is effective against group A Streptococcus
    D. Meropenem is effective against group A Streptococcus
    E. Pseudomonas infection is effectively treated with metronidazole

24. **A 16-year-old girl and her mother visit you to discuss the merits of the HPV vaccine. Which of the following is correct?**
    A. Both HPV vaccinations administered in the UK are quadrivalent
    B. The HPV vaccination can be given in children and adolescents aged 9 to 15 years and adult females aged 16 to 26
    C. HPV vaccinations aim to target HPV 8, 11, 16, and 18
    D. Two prophylactic HPV vaccinations have been developed which aim to avert 90% or more of squamous cell cancers by HPV prevention
    E. The vaccination is a single-dose vaccine largely delivered through secondary schools

25. **A 34-year-old nulliparous woman is found to have premature ovarian failure but wishes to get pregnant. Which treatment would you consider?**
    A. Clomiphene and metformin
    B. Egg donation
    C. Gonadotrophin therapy
    D. Ovarian drilling
    E. Pulsatile gonadotrophin-releasing hormone

26. **A 23-year-old primiparous woman comes to see you at 38 weeks gestation with breech presentation, following a failed external cephalic version. She has come to discuss the benefits of an elective caesarean section versus a normal vaginal breech delivery. What piece of information about the baby should be given to her regarding the benefits of an elective caesarean section?**
    A. Reduces long-term neonatal morbidity
    B. Reduces neonatal mortality
    C. Reduces perinatal mortality and early neonatal morbidity
    D. Reduces perinatal mortality and intermediate term neonatal morbidity
    E. Reduces perinatal mortality and long-term neonatal morbidity

27. **A 36-year-old woman with known toxoplasmosis infection delivers at 38 weeks gestation. What clinical manifestation of toxoplasmosis may be seen in the neonate?**
    A. Cleft lip/palate
    B. Easy bruising
    C. High-pitched cry
    D. Imperforate anus
    E. Jaundice

28. **A 57-year-old woman presents following two episodes of postmenopausal bleeding. What is her risk of endometrial polyps or endometrial hyperplasia?**
    A. 10%
    B. 15%
    C. 20%
    D. 30%
    E. 40%

29. **Regarding statistical analysis, which of the following is true?**
    A. Chi-squared tests are used to compare the difference between two medians
    B. If $p < 0.5$, it is statistically significant
    C. If $p = 0$, this means the chance of something happening is 100%
    D. A test which has 90% sensitivity to predict preterm labour implies that 90% of women going into preterm labour would have an abnormal test result
    E. Type 1 errors occur when the null hypothesis is wrongly accepted

30. **Which one of the following is a normal physiological change in pregnancy?**
    A. Decreased systemic vascular resistance
    B. Increased arterial blood pressure by 10–15 mmHg
    C. Increased arterial pCO_2
    D. Plasma volume increased by up to 20%
    E. Residual capacity is increased by 25%

31. **You are asked to review a 26-year-old woman in antenatal clinic with regard to the impact of her medical history on the duration of second stage in labour. Which one of the following medical conditions requires a shorter second stage?**
    A. Asthma
    B. Knee arthritis
    C. Pre-eclampsia requiring antihypertensive therapy
    D. Presence of ocular chorioretinitis
    E. Spinal cord injury

32. **A 24-year-old woman in her first pregnancy is referred to see you as she has female genital mutilation (FGM). What complication in pregnancy is associated with FGM?**
    A. There is a higher risk of breech presentation
    B. There is a higher risk of foetal growth restriction
    C. There is a higher risk of postpartum haemorrhage
    D. There is a higher risk of prolonged first stage of labour
    E. There is a higher risk of recurrent miscarriage

33. **You are asked to record the POP-Q score for prolapse in a 68-year-old woman. How is point Aa defined?**
    A. It is 3 cm proximal to external urethral meatus
    B. It is 3 cm proximal to the hymen, on the posterior vaginal wall
    C. It is the most distal part of the anterior vaginal wall
    D. It is the most distal part of the posterior vaginal wall
    E. It is the posterior fornix, in those who still have their cervix

34. **A 24-year-old woman presents at six weeks gestation in her first pregnancy. Upon reviewing her medical history, you note that she is taking the drug lithium for psychosis. Which foetal anomaly is this associated with?**
    A. Cardiac defects
    B. Dermatological problems in the neonate
    C. Ebstein's anomaly
    D. Foetal cleft palate
    E. IUGR

35. **Which of the following statements describes the qualities of danazol?**
    A. Danazol has pro-progestogenic activity
    B. Danazol is a synthetic androgenic precursor
    C. Danazol potentiates pituitary gonadotrophin release
    D. Voice changes may occur but are reversible on stopping danazol
    E. Women must use barrier contraception when taking danazol

36. **When you arrive on labour ward for your on-call day, the following women were present with breech presentation. Which patient is most suitable for an ECV today?**

    A. A 20-year-old P0 + 1 woman at 35 + 4 weeks gestation with gestational diabetes with no maternal or foetal complications, attending for steroids

    B. A 24-year-old multiparous woman 39 + 3 weeks with spontaneous ruptured membranes (meconium stained), but not contracting

    C. A 26-year-old nulliparous woman at 39 + 2 weeks gestation, attending for blood pressure check, found to have a breech presentation; blood pressure is currently 124/76, with no symptoms or signs of pre-eclampsia

    D. A 28-year-old P1 + 0 woman at 35 + 4 weeks gestation with previous spontaneous preterm labour at 32 weeks, attending with irregular contractions

    E. A 30-year-old P1 + 3 woman who is 39 + 5 weeks gestation with antepartum haemorrhage three days ago, now settled

37. **A 32-year-old nulliparous woman undergoing IVF enquires about the risk factors for ovarian hyperstimulation syndrome (OHSS). Which one of the following is a risk factor for OHSS?**

    A. History of an endometrioma

    B. IVF cycles where conception does not occur

    C. Maternal age over 40

    D. Women with polycystic ovary syndrome

    E. Women with systemic lupus erythematosus

38. **A 32-year-old primiparous woman books at 12 weeks gestation with a BMI of 55. What management would you advocate?**

    A. Active management of the third stage

    B. Recommend elective caesarean section for women with extreme obesity (BMI > 50)

    C. Recommend epidural analgesia early in labour

    D. Regular cervical length assessment due to the increased risk of preterm labour

    E. Routine episiotomy

39. **You are fast-bleeped to attend a major post-partum haemorrhage on the labour ward. Which of the following statements regarding resuscitation is correct?**

    A. The amount of blood lost at the time of the bleep is over 1,500 ml

    B. Blood transfusion must be started by the time 5 litres of clear fluid have been infused

    C. Crystalloid fluid should be avoided

    D. Four units of fresh frozen plasma should be given if the prothrombin time/activated partial thromboplastin time is above 1.5 times the normal limit

    E. Recombinant activated factor VII (rFVIIa) should be given as early as possible

40. **You are in day surgery reviewing a 29-year-old woman who is about to undergo a laparoscopy. Which of the following statements regarding the safety of laparoscopy in gynaecology is correct?**
    A. Direct trocar insertion has an increased risk of major complications compared to the Hasson technique
    B. Hasson technique is recommended for all patients
    C. The risk of bowel damage is about 4 in 10,000 operations
    D. The risk of damage to major blood vessels is 0.4%
    E. The risk of major vessel injury can be minimized by open (Hasson) technique

41. **Which one of the following is a true finding from the Confidential Enquiries into Maternal Deaths and Morbidity 2018–20?**
    A. 10% fewer women died during childbirth compared to 2017–19
    B. Black women were 3.7 times more likely to die than white women
    C. Two women died from COVID-19
    D. 20% of women died in the postnatal period
    E. Asian women were 3.7 times more likely to die than white women

42. **A 39-year-old multiparous woman presents with a two-year history of mild menorrhagia and worsening urinary frequency. An ultrasound shows a 6 cm submucosal fibroid and 7 cm intramural fibroid. She would prefer to preserve her uterus. What treatment will reduce the size of her fibroids?**
    A. Endometrial ablation
    B. High-dose oral progestogen
    C. Hysterectomy
    D. Tranexamic acid
    E. Uterine artery embolization

43. **A 32-year-old woman is diagnosed to have gestational trophoblastic disease. Her HCG levels revert to normal within six weeks of surgical treatment and she does not fulfil the criteria for further treatment. How long should she be followed-up for?**
    A. Six months from the date of uterine evacuation
    B. Six months from normalization of the HCG level
    C. One year from the pregnancy event
    D. One year from normalization of the HCG level
    E. No further follow-up is required

44. **A 25-year-old woman presents in labour at 39 weeks gestation in her second pregnancy. She had an emergency caesarean section in her first pregnancy following a failed forceps delivery, 11 months ago. She now complains of constant abdominal pain, worsening over the last hour. There are unprovoked prolonged decelerations on the CTG and the baseline has risen from 140 bpm to 160 bpm. Her cervix is 8 cm dilated, with irregular contractions. What is your management plan?**
    A. Category 1 caesarean section
    B. Instrumental delivery in delivery room
    C. Perform foetal blood sampling
    D. Start oxytocin infusion and commence active pushing when contractions re-established
    E. Trial of instrumental delivery in operating theatre

45. **The CMACE report highlights the key infections causing maternal death. Regarding sepsis in pregnancy, which of the following is true?**
    A. *E. Coli* was the most common causative organism
    B. Group A beta haemolytic Streptococcus is a hospital-acquired infection which was the most commonly found organism to cause septic shock
    C. High-dose corticosteroids should be administered
    D. Sepsis was the leading cause of indirect deaths in the 2018–20 triennial report
    E. Septic shock is defined as sepsis with arterial hypotension that is refractory to fluid resuscitation

46. **A 24-year-old woman with a BMI of 38 is diagnosed with polycystic ovary syndrome (PCOS). What complication is associated with PCOS?**
    A. Cataracts
    B. Cervical cancer
    C. Dyslipidaemia
    D. Menorrhagia
    E. Thromboembolism

47. **A 24-year-old primigravid woman presents at 36 weeks of pregnancy with vulval pain and multiple superficial ulcerations on the left labial fold. How will you manage her?**
    A. Administer acyclovir
    B. Admit for analgesia and observation
    C. Induce labour in the next 24 hours
    D. Perform an emergency caesarean section
    E. Take a low vaginal swab and a swab from the ulcer

48. A 16-year-old girl presents with primary amenorrhoea. Which one of the following correlates to the correct diagnosis?

A. An abdominal ultrasound is essential to diagnose an imperforate hymen

B. A FSH level of 45 IU/L indicates ovarian failure

C. If only the FSH level is low, hypothalamic amenorrhoea should be considered

D. Karyotyping should be performed to exclude Kallmann's syndrome

E. A low LH level suggests hypergonadotrophic hypogonadism

49. Regarding lactation, which one of the following drugs is correctly matched to its effect on lactation?

A. Cabergoline suppresses milk production

B. Lactation is stimulated by bromocriptine

C. Metoclopramide is a dopamine agonist and it inhibits lactation

D. Oxytocin stimulates milk production and prolactin stimulates its ejection

E. A rise in progesterone levels stimulates lactation

50. You are counselling a 37-year-old woman and her partner on IVF treatment. Which one of the following is the most important factor in predicting the outcome of fertility treatment?

A. Anti-Müllerian hormone levels

B. Inhibin B and oestradiol level

C. Maternal age

D. Ovarian blood flow

E. Ovarian volume

Extended Matching Questions

Options for Questions 1–5

For each of the following clinical scenarios, choose the most appropriate option from the list provided. Each option may be used once, more than once, or not at all.

A. Acute abdomen
B. Acute appendicitis
C. Acute pelvic inflammatory disease
D. Acute renal failure
E. Acute torsion of ovary
F. Bowel injury at egg collection
G. Critical OHSS
H. Intraperitoneal bleeding
I. Mild OHSS
J. Moderate OHSS
K. Pulmonary embolism
L. Ruptured ectopic
M. Severe OHSS

1. A 28-year-old woman, with a BMI of 34, is a known case of polycystic ovarian syndrome. She is being treated with a clomiphene citrate regimen of 50-mg dose. She is complaining of a bloated abdomen and feels uncomfortable as a result.

2. A 34-year-old woman, with a BMI of 32, underwent an embryo transfer five days ago. She has now been admitted to the acute medical ward with nausea, vomiting, and moderate abdominal pain.

3. A 24-year-old woman, with a BMI of 24, has a high anti-Müllerian hormone (AMH) and had embryo transfer three days ago. She has been admitted to the acute gynaecology ward with clinical ascites and reduced renal output.

4. A 35-year-old woman who had an embryo transfer eight days ago is now complaining of a bloated feeling and an increase in weight of 2 kg. She had a pelvic ultrasound scan reporting an ovarian size >12 cm^2.

5. A 22-year-old woman who is a known case of polycystic ovarian syndrome with a history of OHSS is in her first IVF cycle and is recently undergoing her second treatment cycle. She is day 12 post–embryo transfer. She is complaining of nausea and sudden onset of right-sided abdominal pain following intercourse.

Options for Questions 6–10

For each of the following clinical scenarios, choose the single most likely diagnosis from the list provided. Each option may be used once, more than once, or not at all.

A. Benign intracranial hypertension
B. Cerebral venous thrombosis
C. Cluster-type headache
D. Epilepsy
E. Menstrual-related migraine
F. Migraine with aura
G. Migraine without aura

H. Pre-eclampsia

I. Pseudo-seizures

J. Subarachnoid haemorrhage

K. Tension headache

L. Thrombocytopenic purpura

6. A 24-year-old primigravid woman who is 24 weeks pregnant complains of a pulsating, right-sided headache for 48 hours. This is associated with nausea and vomiting. She also complains of seeing 'flickering lights'.

7. A 32-year-old multiparous woman who is 20 weeks pregnant complains of a pressing bilateral headache for more than ten days.

8. A 20-year-old primigravid woman who is 18 weeks pregnant complains of sharp, left-sided headache, particularly around the eye. This is associated with a red eye and runny nose.

9. A 17-year-old woman has a history of heavy menstrual bleeding since menarche. She complains of a left-sided headache, particularly 2–3 days before her periods.

10. A 38-year-old multiparous woman at 36 weeks of pregnancy presents with history of headaches, vomiting, and photophobia. Her examination has signs of raised intracranial pressure.

Options for Questions 11–15

For each of the following clinical scenarios, choose the single most likely action from the list provided. Each option may be used once, more than once, or not at all.

A. Combined active and passive immunization

B. Confirm primary genital herpes by serological tests

C. Emergency caesarean section

D. HVS for GBS at 36 weeks and if negative no further action

E. HVS every four weeks from 24 weeks of pregnancy and intrapartum benzyl penicillin if positive

F. If she gives a history of having suffered from chickenpox before, no further action is required

G. Intravenous acyclovir before and during labour

H. Neonatal hepatitis B vaccine

I. The neonate should be given neonatal VZIG

J. The neonate should be tested for VZ IgM before initiating any treatment

K. Prophylactic intravenous benzylpenicillin in labour without testing

L. Start immunoglobulins only if serological tests are negative

M. Start immunoglobulins while awaiting serological test results

N. Tocolysis for 24 hours with intravenous acyclovir and then planned caesarean section

O. Treat mother with lamivudine therapy

11. A 29-year-old schoolteacher at eight weeks of pregnancy comes to her GP saying a few children in her class have recently been diagnosed with chickenpox. What will be the GP's next course of action?

12. A 32-year-old woman whose previous pregnancy was complicated by neonatal group-B-streptococcal infection is worried about the same happening in this pregnancy. How will you counsel her?

13. A 26-year-old woman attends the antenatal clinic at 19 weeks of pregnancy. Her antenatal screening bloods show her to have a positive hepatitis B result. Serological screening shows her

to be hepatitis B surface antigen positive, hepatitis E antigen-negative, and anti-Hbe reactive. Her liver function tests are as follows: bilirubin 25 mg/dl, aspartate aminotransferase 96 IU, alanine aminotransferase 70 IU, and alkaline phosphatase 900 IU. What is the most appropriate intervention in preventing mother-to-child transmission?

14. A 26-year-old woman develops chickenpox rash two days after giving birth. Her booking bloods had shown her to be non-immune to varicella. Her baby appears healthy and is breastfeeding. What will be the next step in your management?

15. A 30-year-old woman in her first pregnancy is admitted to labour with ruptured membranes at term. During speculum examination she was found to have vulval lesions highly suggestive of herpetic eruptions. When asked, the patient denied having similar eruptions before. How will you plan her labour?

Options for Questions 16–20

For each of the following clinical scenarios, choose the single most likely treatment from the list provided. Each option may be used once, more than once, or not at all.

    A. Accept infertility

    B. Adoption

    C. Bromocriptine

    D. Clomiphene

    E. Cryopreservation of semen

    F. Donor insemination

    G. Electro-ejaculation for insemination

    H. Gonadotrophin-releasing hormones

    I. ICSI

    J. IVF

    K. Natural intercourse

    L. Ovarian stimulation and IUI

    M. Testicular sperm aspiration

16. A 30-year-old man with Klinefelter syndrome is seen at the infertility clinic accompanied by a female partner with normal investigations.

17. A 35-year-old man with oligo-azoospermia with low FSH, low LH, and low testosterone.

18. A 25-year-old man with spinal cord injury with a normal semen analysis attends the infertility clinic along with his healthy female partner; they have a three-year history of infertility.

19. An 18-year-old man diagnosed with leukaemia requiring chemotherapy therapy.

20. A 35-year-old man with oligo-azoospermia noted to have a first-grade varicocele.

Options for Questions 21–25

For each of the following clinical scenarios, choose the single most likely treatment from the list provided. Each option may be used once, more than once, or not at all.

    A. Adrenaline 1 mg iv every 3–5 minutes

    B. Atropine 3 mg iv once only

    C. Basic life support

    D. Calcium gluconate 10 mg iv

    E. Cardiac pacing

    F. Cardiac shock using a current of 200 joules and repeated as necessary

    G. Dobutamine infusion

H. Emergency caesarean section in operating theatre

I. Hydrocortisone

J. Intralipid

K. Intravenous bicarbonate

L. Intubate and transfer to ITU for ventilation

M. Obstetric ultrasound

N. Perimortem caesarean section in emergency department

O. Steroids to help mature foetal lungs

P. Thrombolysis for massive pulmonary embolism

21. A previously fit, 37-year-old obese primiparous woman attends the emergency department with acute-onset chest pain and some shortness of breath at 32 weeks of gestation. Whilst waiting to be seen, she suddenly collapses on the floor. A junior doctor assesses the patient and on finding no cardiac output, the 'crash team' is summoned and CPR started. The obstetric, anaesthetic, operating theatre, and neonatal team are all alerted. There is no response to CPR at five minutes.

22. A 26-year-old woman who has collapsed upon transfer to the local central delivery unit from a stand-alone birth centre (BC) situated 13 miles away. After an uneventful birth, she sustained approximately 700 ml of blood loss (in the BC) with a partially separated placenta.

23. A 28-year-old nulliparous woman at 30 weeks of pregnancy was admitted to the labour ward with a history of sudden onset of abdominal pain and no bleeding. Her pulse is 120 bpm and her blood pressure is 140/105. Her abdomen seems hard.

24. An 18-year-old nulliparous woman with a previous history of PE had a rapid forceps delivery for acute foetal distress. She sustained a second-degree tear. Local anaesthetic was infiltrated for repair. Her midwife noted that she has suddenly turned blue and has now become unresponsive.

25. A 26-year-old multiparous known asthmatic, now 34 weeks pregnant. She was working in her garden and suddenly started experiencing difficulty breathing. She turned blue and suddenly collapsed.

Options for Questions 26–30

The list of options below refers to the United Kingdom Medical Eligibility Criteria (UKMEC) for contraceptive use. This is a set of agreed norms for providing contraception to women with a range of medical conditions, which may contraindicate one or more contraceptive methods. For each clinical scenario below, choose the single most appropriate UKMEC category from the above list of options. Each option may be used once, more than once, or not at all.

A. Category 1

B. Category 2

C. Category 3

D. Category 4

E. Category 5

F. None of the above

26. A 38-year-old woman is interested in using the combined vaginal ring (CVR) for contraception. She previously used the combined oral contraceptive pill (COC) from age 17 years to age 34 years without any problems. There are no medical illnesses. Her blood pressure is normal and her BMI is 24. She stopped smoking eight months ago, prior to that she smoked 5–10 cigarettes per day.

27. A 30-year-old nulliparous woman requests intrauterine contraception. She has a past medical history of subacute bacterial endocarditis. There are no other medical illnesses.

28. A 42-year-old woman requests the subdermal implant for contraception. Approximately eight years ago she had a mastectomy for an oestrogen receptor positive breast cancer followed by chemotherapy and treatment with tamoxifen. There is no evidence of recurrent disease. She does not have any other medical illnesses.

29. A 25-year-old woman would like to restart combined hormonal contraception (CHC), which she has used without problems in the past. She was diagnosed with gestational trophoblastic disease following a miscarriage three months ago. Her b-HCG levels are gradually declining but are still detectable. She has not been sexually active since the miscarriage.

30. A 24-year-old woman requests the combined transdermal patch for contraception (CTP) and to control her heavy painful periods. She used the COC when she was 17 years with good effect for her periods, but had problems with compliance. She was diagnosed with essential hypertension two years ago. Her blood pressure is well controlled on antihypertensive medication. There are no other illnesses. Her BMI is 35. She smokes 5–10 cigarettes per day.

Options for Questions 31–36

For each of the following questions, choose the single most appropriate staging option from those provided. Each option may be used once, more than once, or not at all.

A. Stage 1A
B. Stage 1B
C. Stage 2
D. Stage 3A1
E. Stage 3A2
F. Stage 3B1
G. Stage 3B2
H. Stage 3C
I. Stage 4A1
J. Stage 4A2
K. Stage 4B

31. Squamous carcinoma of the vulva which is 1 cm in diameter with a solitary nodal mass in the left internal iliac region suggesting metastasis.

32. A single 1.8 cm midline vulval lesion at the forchette with 0.9-mm stromal invasion. There are no palpable lymph nodes.

33. A 4 cm midline vulval tumour invading 3 mm into the lower urethra.

34. A 4 cm midline vulval tumour invading 3 mm into underlying stroma only.

35. A 2.5 cm right vulval mass with one left inguinofemoral node metastasis of 5 mm diameter.

36. A 2.5 cm right vulval mass with two left inguinofemoral node metastases of 5 mm diameter.

Options for Questions 37–42

For each of the following symptomatic postmenopausal women, select the most appropriate single therapy. Each option may be used once, more than once, or not at all.

A. Alendronic acid
B. Insertion of levonorgestrel-containing IUS
C. Local vaginal oestrogen therapy
D. Medroxy progesterone acetate
E. Oral combined cyclical hormone replacement therapy

F. Oral phytoestrogens

G. Raloxifen

H. Selective serotonin reuptake inhibitor (SSRI) antidepressants

I. Sildenafil citrate

J. Testosterone supplementation with systemic HRT

K. Tibolone

L. Transdermal oestrogen-only HRT

37. A 57-year-old woman suffering from severe menopausal vasomotor and lower genital tract symptoms; her last period was 12 months ago and she has known large uterine fibroids.

38. A 56-year-old woman with a history of breast cancer, on aromatase inhibitors, with a six-month history of distressing night sweats.

39. A 58-year-old woman who has had a hysterectomy with diagnosed hypoactive sexual desire disorder (HSDD).

40. A 65-year-old nulliparous woman (normal BMI) with a history of breast cancer, now presenting with osteoporosis.

41. A 30-year-old nulliparous woman has been diagnosed with severe endometriosis. She has been commenced on long-term LHRH-A treatment.

42. A 42-year-old multiparous woman with a history of cervical carcinoma, treated with surgery and radiotherapy. She is now complaining of dyspareunia.

Options for Questions 43–47

For each of the following options, choose the single most appropriate definition from the list provided. Each option may be used once, more than once, or not at all.

A. Clinical audit

B. Clinical effectiveness

C. Clinical governance

D. Education and training

E. Justice

F. Openness

G. Patient and public involvement

H. Research and development

I. Risk management

J. Staffing and staff management

K. Using information and IT

43. A measure of the extent to which a particular intervention works.

44. Processes which are open to public scrutiny, while respecting individual patient and practitioner confidentiality, and which can be justified openly.

45. A framework through which NHS organizations are accountable for continually improving the quality of their services and safeguarding high standards of care by creating an environment in which excellence in clinical care will flourish.

46. The review of clinical performance, the refining of clinical practice as a result and the measurement of performance against agreed standards—a cyclical process of improving the quality of clinical care.

47. The identification, assessment, and prioritization of risks, followed by coordinated and economical application of resources to minimize, monitor, and control the probability and/or impact of unfortunate events.

Options for Questions 48–50

For each of the following clinical scenarios, choose the single most appropriate management option. Each option may be used once, more than once, or not at all.

A. Amytryptiline
B. Anterior colporrhaphy
C. Artificial urinary sphincter
D. Augmentation cystoplasty
E. Botulinum A toxin
F. Cimetidine
G. Colposuspension (Burch)
H. Intraurethral NASHA/DX copolymer injection
I. Needle suspension
J. Rectus fascia pubovaginal sling
K. Sacral neuromodulation
L. TOT
M. TVT
N. Urinary diversion

48. An 83-year-old woman in poor medical health with urodynamic stress incontinence and normal voiding parameters.

49. A 44-year-old woman with urge incontinence and severe detrusor overactivity on urodynamic assessment. This is unresponsive to conservative therapy and anticholinergic medications.

50. A 56-year-old woman with urodynamic stress incontinence and no previous surgery; her family is complete and there is no prolapse on examination.

paper
2

ANSWERS

Single Best Answers

1. D. Between 5 and 14 days postoperatively

Ureterovaginal or vesicovaginal fistulae are seen in under 2% of women undergoing radical hysterectomy and usually present between 5 and 14 days postoperatively.

Hadwin R, Petts G, Olaitan A. Treatment related morbidity in gynaecological cancers. *TOG* 2010;12:79–86.

Reed NS, Sadozye AH. Update on radiotherapy in gynaecological malignancies. *TOG* 2017; 19(1):29–36.

Reed NS, Sadozye AH. Update on chemotherapy in gynaecological cancers. *TOG* 2016;18(3):182–8.

2. E. Systemic lupus erythematosus (SLE)

Patients with APS only have similar clinical profiles to those who have APS and SLE, but features such as heart valve disorders, low C4 counts, neutropenia, and haemolytic anaemias are more commonly seen in SLE.

Myers B, Pavord S. Diagnosis and management of antiphospholipid syndrome in pregnancy. *TOG* 2011;13:15–21.

3. A. Copper intrauterine device

Ulipristal acetate is a progesterone receptor modulator which can be administered within five days of the earliest episode of unprotected sexual intercourse, regardless of the number of coital acts within those days. However, it is contraindicated in poorly controlled asthma as well as severe hepatic disease. The copper intrauterine device should therefore be prescribed.

Bhathena R, Guillebaud J. Postcoital contraception. *TOG* 2011;13:29–34.

4. E. Up to 27 in 100 women

In women with placenta praevia, the risk of an emergency hysterectomy is up to 11 in 100 women. However, if she has had a previous caesarean section, her risk of an emergency hysterectomy increases up to 27 in 100 women.

RCOG Consent Advice 12. Caesarean section for placenta praevia; January 2011.

5. E. Mirena intrauterine system

The COC pill is contraindicated in obese smokers over the age of 35. The Mirena intrauterine system is licensed for treatment of menorrhagia but can also alleviate dysmenorrhoea.

NICE Clinical Guideline 88. Heavy menstrual bleeding: assessment and management; 2018.

6. B. Breast cancer

Breast cancer is the most common malignancy associated with pregnancy, with an incidence of approximately 1 in 3,000 pregnancies.

Padmagirison R, Gajjar K, Spencer C. Management of breast cancer during pregnancy. *TOG* 2010;12:186–92.

RCOG Green-top Guideline 12. Pregnancy and breast cancer; March 2011.

7. B. Adrenal tumour

A very high testosterone level (i.e. over 2 ng/ml) increases the likelihood of cancer and an elevated dehydroepiandrosterone sulphate level suggests an adrenal source. In addition, a pelvic ultrasound has been normal.

Swingler R, Awala A, Gordon U. Hirsutism in young women. *TOG* 2009;11:101–7.

8. A. Foetal talipes

Amniocentesis before 14 weeks of gestation has a higher foetal loss rate and increased risk of foetal talipes. It is also associated with a higher respiratory morbidity.

RCOG Green-top Guideline 8. Amniocentesis and chorionic villus sampling; Oct 2021.

9. C. The risk of miscarriage is unchanged when compared to the general population

The median survival for women with cystic fibrosis is 31 years. Fertility and the risk of miscarriage are unchanged. Whilst there is an increased risk of prematurity, there is no association with foetal growth restriction or congenital malformations.

Ashcroft, A, Chapman, SJ, Mackillop, L. The outcome of pregnancy in women with cystic fibrosis: a UK population based descriptive study. *BJOG* 2020;127:16961703.

10. D. Previous history of placental abruption

Whilst all are risk factors for placental abruption, the most predictive factor for placental abruption is a previous history of placental abruption. Other risk factors include assisted conception techniques, maternal thrombophilias, smoking, cocaine use, and first-trimester bleeding.

RCOG Green-top Guideline 63. Antepartum haemorrhage; November 2011.

11. E. Uterovaginal agenesis

Uterovaginal agenesis, also known as Mayer–Rokitansky–Kuster–Hauser syndrome is rare, usually presenting during the teenage years with primary amenorrhoea in the presence of normal secondary sexual characteristics. As the ovaries are normal, puberty occurs at the expected time in the expected order. Approximately 40% of these women will have renal tract abnormalities.

Demonds DK, Rose GL. Outflow tract disorders of the female genital tract. *TOG* 2013;15:11–17.

12. E. Prescribe thromboprophylaxis

Management involves keeping the patient warm, administering oxygen, and prescribing analgesia. However, pethidine is generally less effective in managing sickle-cell-related pain. As both sickle cell disease and pregnancy are recognized risk factors for venous thromboembolism, thromboprophylactic measures should be prescribed upon admission.

British Society of Haematology Guideline/RCOG Green-top Guideline 61. Guidelines for the management of sickle cell disease in pregnancy; August 2021.

Eissa A, Tuck S. Sickle cell disease and beta-thalassaemia major in pregnancy. *TOG* 2013;15:71–8.

13. C. Review the evidence of training and continuing professional development in the department

The National Ultrasound Steering Group published recommendations on quality assurance on ultrasound provision in 2008. In relation to governance and standards, this includes evidence of training, continuing professional development of operators, audit, and adverse incident reporting.

National Ultrasound Steering Group. Ultrasound clinical governance; 2008.

14. B. Sentinel node assessment using radioisotope scintigraphy can be performed in pregnancy

Surgical treatment including loco-regional clearance or mastectomy can be undertaken in all trimesters. Reconstruction should be delayed to avoid prolonged anaesthesia and to allow optimal symmetrization of the breasts after delivery. Sentinel node assessment using radioisotope scintigraphy does not cause significant uterine radiation. Systemic chemotherapy is contraindicated in the first trimester because of a high rate of foetal abnormality, but is safe from the second trimester and should be offered according to protocols. Tamoxifen and trastuzumab are contraindicated in pregnancy and should not be used.

RCOG Green-top Guideline 12. Pregnancy and breast cancer; 2011.

15. B. HIV-positive women who develop chickenpox in pregnancy should be referred to hospital

VZV is a DNA virus of the herpes family. It is highly contagious and transmitted via respiratory droplets and by direct personal contact with vesicle fluid or indirectly via fomites. VZV is infectious 48 hours before the rash appears and continues to be infectious until the vesicles crust over. The vesicles usually have crusted over within five days. The virus remains dormant in sensory nerve root ganglia. It can be reactivated to cause a vesicular erythematous skin rash in a dermatomal distribution, manifesting as shingles. VZIG has no therapeutic benefit once chickenpox has developed. Women with significant immunosuppression, chest symptoms, a dense or haemorrhagic rash, or neurological symptoms should be referred to hospital.

RCOG Green-top Guideline No 13. Chickenpox in pregnancy; January 2015.

16. D. Women with PCOS have a high prevalence of impaired glucose tolerance test and type 2 diabetes mellitus compared to the general population

Women with PCOS may have a higher cardiovascular risk than weight-matched controls with normal ovarian function. They have increased cardiovascular risk factors such as obesity, hyperandrogenism, hyperlipidaemia, and hyperinsulinaemia. An abnormal lipid profile mainly consists of raised triglycerides, and total and low-density lipoprotein cholesterol. All these are the bad quality lipids and all these risk factors in young PCOS women increase the risk of developing accelerated atherosclerosis resulting in myocardial infarction. In PCOS women, there is an increased incidence of impaired glucose tolerance test and later type 2 diabetes. As there is hyperinsulinaemia with tissue resistance, this leads to abnormal glucose metabolism. For patients with evidence of clinical hyperandrogenism, such as male type of baldness, beard, excessive hair on the body with male pattern, and with a total serum testosterone level of more than 5 nmol/L, it is advisable to rule out androgen-secreting tumours, and 17-hydroxyprogesterone should be sampled. Blood pressure ≥140/90 mmHg not responding to healthy lifestyle changes warrants drug therapy and regular follow-up to minimize other risk factors.

RCOG Green-top Guideline 33. Long-term consequences of polycystic ovary syndrome; 2014.

17. D. Isoniazid and rifampicin

The diagnosis here is tuberculosis. Common presenting symptoms include cough, shortness of breath, night sweats, and wheeze. Investigations include the Mantoux skin test, chest X-ray, culture from sputum or gastric fluid, and other imaging modalities such as CT of chest. Treatment of TB usually includes isoniazid, rifampicin, and pyridoxine.

Public Health England (2019). Pregnancy and tuberculosis (TB) Information for clinicians. [online] Available at: https://assets.publishing.service.gov.uk/government/uploads/system/uploads/attachment_data/file/851836/RA_Pregnancy_TB_Clinicians.pdf.

18. B. It may be achieved via the vaginoscopic route

With pre-procedure analgesia and modern scopes, success rates with nulliparous women are high. With good irrigation a good view of the cavity can be achieved. These are all procedures that should be performed in outpatients in a 'see and treat' environment. Vaginoscopy achieves a 'no touch' instrumentation of the cervix which is associated with less pain. Due to the risks of general anaesthetic, outpatient hysteroscopy should be considered the first-line diagnostic approach.

BSGE/RCOG Green-top Guideline 59: Best Practice in outpatient hysteroscopy; March 2011.

19. E. Transabdominal cerclage can be performed in early pregnancy

Cerclage is not recommended for ultrasound-identified funnelling of the cervix in the absence of cervical shortening to 25 mm or less. A transabdominal cerclage is usually inserted following an unsuccessful vaginal cerclage or extensive cervical surgery. Cerclage is not recommended in women on the basis of a history of previous cervical cone biopsy alone. Transabdominal cerclage can be performed preconceptually or in early pregnancy. Contraindications to cerclage insertion do include PPROM.

Shennan AH, Story L; the Royal College of Obstetricians and Gynaecologists. Cervical cerclage. *BJOG* 2022;129:1178–210.

20. D. Osteoporosis is confirmed with a T score of −2.5 on DEXA scan

Combined HRT can be given to women who have had BSO for *BRCA* mutation. Clonidine is used to treat hot flushes and night sweats.

NICE Guideline 23. Menopause: diagnosis and management; November 2015.

RCOG Scientific Paper 6. Alternatives to HRT for the management of symptoms of the menopause; 2010.

21. D. Neonatal hyperthyroidism

Uncontrolled hyperthyroidism increases the risk of IUGR, preterm labour, and foetal and neonatal death. Rarely, autoantibodies can cross the placenta and cause neonatal hyperthyroidism.

Nelson-Piercy C. *Handbook of obstetric medicine*. Boca Raton: CRC Press; 2021.

22. D. Request an MRI and refer to a gynaecology oncologist

For women with a high risk of cancer (RMI > 250), management should occur in a cancer centre with full staging. The RMI is based on the ultrasound features, menopausal status, and CA125 level.

RCOG Green-top Guideline 34. The management of ovarian cysts in postmenopausal women; 2016.

23. D. Meropenem is effective against group A Streptococcus

Co-amoxiclav does not treat MRSA. Some microbiologists prefer to limit routine use as it can predispose to MRSA colonization. Vancomycin and teicoplanin are important antibiotics used to treat MRSA. Meropenem is an important broad-spectrum antibiotic effective against many groups of bacteria (excluding MRSA). Clindamycin is effective against most anaerobes, along with many Gram-positive bacteria. Pseudomonas is a Gram-negative bacteria, and therefore often sensitive to gentamicin. Metronidazole is effective against anaerobes. Gentamicin is effective against Gram-negative bacteria and Staphylococcus, but not Streptococci bacteria. Antibiotics effective against group A Streptococcus include ampicillin, co-amoxiclav, cefuroxime, meropenem, and tazocin.

RCOG Green-top Guideline 64b. Bacterial sepsis following pregnancy, Appendix IV; 2012.

24. B. HPV vaccination can be given in children and adolescents aged 9 to 15 years and adult females aged 16 to 26

Two prophylactic HPV vaccinations have been developed, which aim to avert 70% or more of squamous cell cancers by HPV prevention. Gardasil is a quadrivalent vaccine; Cervarix is bivalent. HPV vaccination can be given in children and adolescents aged 9 to 15 years and adult females aged 16 to 26. The vaccination consists of three injections which should ideally be given over a period of six months, although they can be given over a period of 12 months. Cervarix is bivalent and protects only against HPV types 16 and 18, whilst Gardasil protects against HPV 6, 11, 16, and 18.

British Society for Colposcopy and Cervical Pathology. Available at: https://www.bsccp.org.uk

25. B. Egg donation

Hypothalamic-pituitary-ovarian dysfunction (PCOS) is best managed with weight reduction, clomiphene citrate, or clomiphene citrate plus metformin as first-line therapy. When the first-line therapy fails, then ovarian drilling or clomiphene plus metformin may be considered, or gonadotrophin therapy. In PCOS gonadotrophins should not be combined with gonadotrophin-releasing hormone agonists concomitantly; this does not improve pregnancy rate but is associated with an increased risk of ovarian hyperstimulation. The effectiveness of pulsatile gonadotrophin-releasing hormone in women with clomiphene-resistant PCOS is uncertain and is not recommended in clinical practice. In ovarian failure, the ovaries are non-functional due to radiation exposure, cancer therapy, or familial history; the only way for pregnancy is egg donation.

NICE Clinical Guideline 156. Fertility problems: assessment and treatment; 2013.

26. C. Reduces perinatal mortality and early neonatal morbidity

Women should be informed that planned caesarean section carries a reduced perinatal mortality and early neonatal morbidity for babies with breech presentation at term when compared to a planned vaginal delivery. There is no evidence that the long-term health of babies with breech presentation delivered at term is influenced by the mode of delivery.

RCOG Green-top Guideline 20a. External cephalic version and reducing the incidence of breech presentation; 2017.

27. E. Jaundice

Toxoplasmosis mainly affects the central nervous system and eyes, leading to chorioretinitis and blindness. Ventriculomegaly, hydrocephalus, and convulsions may be seen, with learning difficulties seen later on in life. Other manifestations include anaemia, rash, pneumonitis, hepatosplenomegaly, and jaundice.

To M, Kidd M, Maxwell D. Prenatal diagnosis and management of fetal infections. *TOG* 2009;11:108–16.

28. E. 40%

Patients with postmenopausal bleeding have a 10–15% risk of endometrial carcinoma, but the prevalence of endometrial polyps or hyperplasia is estimated to be 40%.

Bakour S, Timmermans A, Willem B, Khan K. Management of women with post-menopausal bleeding: evidence-based review. *TOG* 2012;14:243–9.

BSGE/RCOG Green-top Guideline No. 67. Management of endometrial hyperplasia; 2016.

29. **D.** A test which has 90% sensitivity to predict preterm labour implies that 90% of women going into preterm labour would have an abnormal test result

The p value is found only at the end of a study and is usually fixed at 0.05 or 5%. The smaller the p value, the stronger the evidence that the findings are significant. A type 1 error occurs if a correct hypothesis is rejected. A type 2 error occurs when a wrong hypothesis is accepted and is more commonly seen when the sample size is small. Statistical significance is generally achieved when $p < 0.05$. Chi-squared tests are used to compare distributions and depend on the observed and expected results only. Sensitivity is the proportion of all cases which have an abnormal test result. By comparison, specificity is defined as the proportion of cases which do *not* have an abnormality with a normal test result.

Luesley DM, Kilby MD. *Obstetrics & gynaecology: an evidence-based text for the MRCOG.* Boca Raton: CRC Press; 2016.

30. **A.** Decreased systemic vascular resistance

Plasma volume is increased by up to 40%. Systemic vascular resistance is decreased whilst arterial blood pressure decreases by 10–15 mmHg. Arterial PCO_2 is decreased due to the effect of progesterone on respiratory drive. This is due to the splinting of the diaphragm by the gravid uterus.

RCOG. Green-top Guideline 56. Maternal collapse in pregnancy and the puerperium; 2019.

31. **E.** Spinal cord injury

Maternal indications to decrease the length and impact of the second stage of labour on medical conditions include hypertensive crises, significant cardiac disease, myasthenia gravis, proliferative retinopathy, and spinal cord injury patients who are at risk of autonomic dysreflexia.

RCOG Green-top Guideline 26. Assisted vaginal birth; Jan. 2020.

32. **C.** There is a higher risk of post-partum haemorrhage

FGM does not increase pregnancy-related risks as genital mutilation procedures involve anatomical damage to the vaginal and vulval tissue, leading to scarring and reduced stretchability of the tissue during the second stage. There is an increased risk of PPH.

RCOG Green-top Guideline 53. Female Genital Mutilation and its management; July 2015.

33. **A.** It is 3 cm proximal to the external urethral meatus

Point Ba is the most distal part of the anterior vaginal wall. Point Ap is 3 cm proximal to the hymen, on the posterior vaginal wall. Point Bp is the most distal part of the posterior vaginal wall. Point C is most distal part of the cervix, or vaginal vault; Point D is the posterior fornix, in those who still have their cervix.

NICE Guideline 123. Urinary incontinence and pelvic organ prolapse in women: management; April 2019

34. **C.** Ebstein's anomaly

Lithium is recognized to cause foetal heart defects, in particular Ebstein's anomaly. Consideration should be given to discontinuing the drug and switching to an alternative antipsychotic if necessary, or stopping as soon as pregnancy is confirmed and restarting in the second trimester. Withdrawal of lithium should be gradual over four weeks. The SSRI paroxetine has been shown to cause foetal heart defects if taken in the first trimester. Any woman planning a pregnancy or with an unplanned pregnancy should be advised to stop taking this drug. Lamotrigine is known to cause dermatological problems (notably Stevens–Johnson syndrome) in the neonate if taken whilst breastfeeding.

Carbamazepine is recognized to cause major foetal malformations such as neural tube, cardiac, and gastrointestinal defects.

NICE Clinical Guideline 192. Antenatal and postnatal mental health: clinical management and service guidance; 2014.

RCOG Good Practice Guideline No. 14. Management of women with mental health issues during pregnancy and the postnatal period; June 2011

35. E. Women must use barrier contraception when taking danazol

Danazol is a synthetic androgenic preparation which inhibits pituitary gonadotrophin release. It may cause irreversible voice changes and virilizes female foetuses.

RCOG Green-top Guideline No.48. Management of premenstrual syndrome. Feb 2017.

36. C. A 26-year-old nulliparous woman at 39 + 2 weeks, attending for a blood pressure check, was found to have a breech presentation; blood pressure is currently 124/76, with no symptoms or signs of pre-eclampsia

Preterm gestation, SROM, and a recent history of antepartum haemorrhage are relative contraindications to ECV.

RCOG Green-top Guideline 20a. External cephalic version and reducing the incidence of breech presentation; 2017.

37. D. Women with polycystic ovary syndrome

OHSS is a systemic disease resulting from vasoactive products released by hyperstimulated ovaries. Increased vascular permeability leads to fluid leakage from the vasculature. It is common to have mild OHSS in IVF cycles (33%) while the moderate to severe form is rare and accounts for 3–8% of IVF cycles.

RCOG Green-top Guideline 5. The management of ovarian hyperstimulation syndrome; 2016.

38. A. Active management of the third stage

The risk of spontaneous preterm labour is lower in obese women. A high pre-pregnancy BMI is associated with a longer gestation at delivery. This has led to the higher rate of induction of labour in obese women. CMACE recommended that in the absence of obstetric or medical indications for caesarean section, vaginal delivery should be encouraged for obese women. Although a midline subumbilical incision potentially offers easier access, the low transverse incision is associated with lower postoperative pain and improved cosmetic effect. The incidence of post-partum haemorrhage is increased in obese women, even after a normal vaginal delivery.

RCOG Green-top Guideline No.72. Care of women with obesity in pregnancy; November 2018.

39. D. Four units of fresh frozen plasma should be given if the prothrombin time/activated partial thromboplastin time is above 1.5 times the normal limit

Major post-partum haemorrhage is defined as blood loss over 1,000 ml and bleeding is continuing or when there is clinical shock. Until blood is available, the initial fluid resuscitation involves infusion of up to 3.5 litres of warmed crystalloid Hartmann's solution (2 litres) and/or colloid (1–2 litres) as rapidly as required. Whilst recombinant activated factor VII (rFVIIa) is known to be effective in controlling bleeding, it should only be used as an adjuvant to standard treatment measures. Four units of fresh frozen plasma should be given for every six units of red cells or if the prothrombin time/activated partial thromboplastin time >1.5 × normal (12–15 ml/kg or total of 1 litre). Blood transfusion must be started by the time 3.5 litres of clear fluid have been infused. This is because blood is required to restore oxygen-carrying capacity. If cross-matched blood is still not available by the time 3.5 litres of fluid have been infused, Group O Rh (D) negative blood should be considered to minimize the risk of a mismatched transfusion.

RCOG Green-top Guideline 47. Blood transfusion in obstetrics; 2015.

RCOG Green-top Guideline 52. Prevention and management of postpartum haemorrhage; 2016.

40. C. The risk of bowel damage is about 4 in 10,000 operations

The risk of bowel injury is 0.4 in 1,000. The risk of major blood vessel damage is 0.2 in 1,000. There is no evidence that the Hasson technique reduces the risk of blood vessel damage. There is no evidence to suggest a higher risk of complications from using direct entry in terms of major complications. The Hasson technique is recommended for both morbidly obese patients and very thin patients.

British Society for Gynaecological Endoscopy. Available at: https://www.bsge.org.uk/guidelines/

41. B. Black women were 3.7 times more likely to die than white women

229 women died during childbirth or up to 6 weeks after in 2018–20. 24% more women died during childbirth compared to figures from the last report. 9 women died from COVID-19. Black women were 3.7 times more likely to die than white women, and Asian women were 1.8 times more likely to die than white women. In 2020, women were three times more likely to die by suicide during or up to six weeks after the end of pregnancy compared to the last report.

Centre for Maternal and Child Enquiries. Lessons learned to inform maternity care from the UK and Ireland Confidential Enquiries into Maternal Deaths and Morbidity 2018–20.

42. E. Uterine artery embolization

Tranexamic acid, high-dose oral progestogens, and endometrial ablation have no effect on the size of fibroid. Hysterectomy is a definitive treatment for fibroids and heavy menstrual bleeding but does not preserve the uterus. Uterine artery embolization shrinks fibroid size by approximately 50%.

NICE Clinical Guideline 88. Heavy menstrual bleeding: assessment and management; 2018.

43. A. Six months from the date of uterine evacuation

Follow-up after gestational trophoblastic disease depends on the individual patient. If HCG has normalized within 56 days of the pregnancy event, then follow-up will be for six months from the date of uterine evacuation. If HCG does not revert to normal levels within 56 days of the pregnancy event, follow-up should be continued for six months from normalization of the HCG level.

RCOG Green-top Guideline 38. Management of Gestational trophoblastic disease; 2020.

44. A. Category 1 caesarean section

Women with a prior history of lower-segment transverse caesarean section have a 0.5% risk of uterine rupture when attempting vaginal birth. Signs and symptoms of uterine rupture include an abnormal cardiotocograph, which is seen in 55–87% of cases. Constant lower abdominal pain which persists between the uterine contractions is a worrying sign. Furthermore, a rise in maternal pulse and fall in blood pressure may be a sign of an impending scar dehiscence. Management should be immediate delivery.

RCOG Green-top Guideline 45. Birth after previous caesarean birth; 2015.

45. E. Septic shock is defined as sepsis with arterial hypotension that is refractory to fluid resuscitation

The use of high-dose corticosteroid therapy no longer has a place in the management of sepsis, however severe. Cardiac diseases were the leading cause of indirect deaths, and VTE being the leading cause of direct deaths, in the 2018–20 triennial report. Septic shock is associated with arterial hypotension that is refractory to fluid resuscitation. Hypotension is the result of loss of vasomotor tone causing arterial vasodilatation along with reduced cardiac output because of myocardial depression, and there is also increased vascular permeability so that fluid leaks into the extravascular compartment. Group A beta haemolytic *Streptococcus* is a community-acquired infection.

Centre for Maternal and Child Enquiries. Lessons learned to inform maternity care from the UK and Ireland Confidential Enquiries into Maternal Deaths and Morbidity 2018–20.

46. C. Dyslipidaemia

Women with PCOS have a higher risk of hypertension, dyslipidaemia, impaired glucose tolerance, NIDDM, and hyperinsulinaemia. Evidence suggests that insulin resistance may be a causative factor in sleep apnoea. Whilst this woman is at higher risk of thromboembolism, her BMI is an independent risk factor associated with this rather than a direct association with PCOS.

RCOG Green-top Guideline 33. Long-term consequences of polycystic ovary syndrome; 2014.

47. A. Administer acyclovir

For acute vulval ulcerations, treatment with acyclovir should be commenced. Acyclovir in pregnancy is generally safe, although not licensed. This should be discussed with the patient. Nucleic acid tests are widely available and give fast results, within hours when needed. If this is a primary attack, elective caesarean delivery may be considered. Otherwise, there is no indication for intervention at this stage. Vaginal delivery in mothers who had previous attacks and developed antibodies may be considered. There is no indication to induce delivery due to vulval ulcerations.

BASHH/ RCOG. Management of genital herpes in pregnancy; 2014.

48. B. A FSH level of 45 IU/L indicates ovarian failure

A low LH level suggests hypogonadotrophic hypogonadism. A high FSH (over 40 IU/L) indicates ovarian failure. If both FSH and LH are low, hypothalamic amenorrhoea or constitutionally delayed puberty should be considered. Karyotyping should be performed to exclude Turner's syndrome; Kallmann's syndrome is not a genetic disorder. Imaging is essential to check the uterus and ovaries are normal, whilst examination inspects the vagina and appearance of the cervix.

NICE Guideline 156. Fertility problems: assessment and treatment; 2013.

49. A. Cabergoline suppresses milk production

Cabergoline is often given to suppress milk production in women who have experienced an intrauterine death or stillbirth. Bromocriptine is a dopamine receptor agonist that inhibits prolactin production and is therefore used to inhibit lactation. Metoclopramide is a dopamine antagonist, increasing prolactin production which stimulates lactation. High levels of sex hormones in pregnancy prevent milk production. Cessation of placental progesterone synthesis at delivery triggers lactation. Conversely, if oestrogens are administered whilst breastfeeding, milk production falls. Prolactin stimulates milk production and oxytocin stimulates its ejection.

Luesley DM, Kilby MD. *Obstetrics & gynaecology: an evidence-based text for the MRCOG.* Boca Raton: CRC Press; 2016.

50. C. Maternal age

Despite advances in reproductive medicine, maternal age is still the most important initial predictor of success for conception both in natural cycles and IVF cycles. With increasing maternal age the low success rate for pregnancies should be discussed with patients rather than giving false reassurance. Anti-Müllerian hormone is widely used in clinical practice to predict the outcome of ovarian response to stimulation in IVF cycles. A level of ≥25.0 pmol/L is suggestive of high response while ≤5.4 pmol/L is predictive of a low response to gonadotrophin ovarian stimulation. FSH of 4 IU/L predicts a high response and greater than 8.9 IU/L predicts a low response. These can be used in combination or in groups to predict the outcome of fertility treatment, but not individually, as there is no evidence in the literature that any one of these will predict the infertility treatment outcome.

NICE Guideline 156. Fertility problems: assessment and treatment; 2013.

Extended Matching Questions

Answers for Questions 1–5

1. I; 2. J; 3. G; 4. M; 5. E

1. A case of mild ovarian hyperstimulation manifested by abdominal bloating, abdominal pain, and ovaries usually less than 8 cm in size.

2. This is a case of moderate OHSS manifested by moderate abdominal pain, nausea, and vomiting, with ultrasound evidence of ascites. Ovarian size is usually between 8 and 12 cm.

3. It is a critical OHSS manifested by tense ascites or large hydrothorax. Haematocrit is usually >55% with evidence of oligo-anuria, white cell count >25,000. These patients are at increased risk of thromboembolism and acute respiratory distress. It is important to recognize that very high levels of AMH are risk factors for critical OHSS.

4. This is a case of severe OHSS, usually presenting with clinical ascites, oliguria, haematocrit >45%, hypoproteinaemia, and ovarian size usually >12 cm.

5. Large hyperstimulated ovaries are at increased risk of torsion and for that reason patients are advised to refrain from sexual intercourse and strenuous exercise. Torsion should always be considered if there is a sudden change or increase in pain, particularly if it is unilateral or associated with leucocytosis, anaemia, and nausea. Ultrasound scan can sometimes be helpful in making a diagnosis as it will demonstrate an increase in size of the ovary with changes to colour Doppler flow in the supplying blood vessels.

RCOG Green-top Guideline 5. The management of ovarian hyperstimulation syndrome; 2016.

Answers for Questions 6–10

6. F; 7. K; 8. C; 9. E; 10. B

6. Migraine may present with or without aura. It may be unilateral or bilateral but is pulsatile in nature. It may be aggravated by routine activities of daily living. Typical aura symptoms include visual symptoms such as flickering lights, spots or lines, and/or partial loss of vision; sensory symptoms such as numbness and/or pins and needles; and/or speech disturbance.

7. A tension headache is usually bilateral, pressing (non-pulsatile), and lasts for 30 minutes (continuous). It may be episodic (occurring fewer than 15 times per month) or chronic (occurring more than 15 times per month, for at least three months).

8. A cluster headache is usually unilateral (around the eye, above the eye, and along the side of the head/face). It is associated with red eye and/or runny nose/nasal congestion.

9. Menstrual-related migraine usually presents 2–3 days before the menstrual cycle. It may have other features of migraine as described previously. A headache diary is recommended for at least two menstrual cycles to reach the diagnosis.

10. The incidence of cerebral venous thrombosis is 1 in 10,000 and is associated with high mortality rates. The majority of cases are seen in pregnant or puerperal women. It should be differentiated from severe pre-eclampsia (as no blood pressure readings have been given). Signs of raised intracranial pressure are suggestive of this diagnosis.

NICE Clinical Guideline 150. Headaches in over 12s: diagnosis and management; 2021.

Answers for Questions 11–15

11. F; 12. K; 13. H; 14. I; 15. C

11. Previous history of exposure to chickenpox has conferred lifelong immunity.

12. Previous history of neonatal infection with group B Streptococcus infection is a valid indication to provide prophylaxis during labour even though a high vaginal swab may be negative.

13. There is a high risk of vertical transmission of hepatitis B to the baby, therefore neonatal hepatitis B immunization is recommended.

14. This baby is at high risk of vertical transmission and therefore should be given neonatal VZIG. There are serious consequences for the baby if not adequately protected.

15. Vaginal herpetic lesions increase vertical transmission risk to the baby during vaginal birth. An emergency caesarean section is indicated.

NICE Guideline 201. Antenatal care; 2021.

Answers for Questions 16–20

16. F; 17. H; 18. J; 19. E; 20. I

16. Patients with Klinefelter syndrome have small testes and are totally azoospermic. There is no case for ICSI in these patients. Management in this case is donor insemination or adoption.

17. This endocrine profile essentially shows hypogonadotrophic hypogonadism. The first option would be to go for gonadotrophin-releasing hormone to see if he responds well.

18. This question does not say how the sample was retrieved. If normal intercourse is possible and he can produce a good semen sample, then IVF should be considered. However, in those patients where ejaculation is not possible naturally, then electro-ejaculation for intrauterine insemination will be appropriate.

19. Chemotherapy can adversely affect spermatogenesis. It is important to cryopreserve his semen sample which can be used later on for his future partner's infertility treatment.

20. Oligo-azoospermia is defined as a count of <5 million per ml and sperm motility of 15%. The literature is rather controversial as to whether treatment of first-grade varicocele will improve sperm function. The couple should be offered ICSI.

NICE Clinical Guideline 156. Fertility problems: assessment and treatment; 2013.

Answers for Questions 21–25

21. N; 22. B; 23. M; 24. J; 25. C

21. The most likely reason for cardiac arrest in the first case was massive pulmonary embolism. If, after five minutes of effective CPR, resuscitation has not been successful, a perimortem caesarean section should be performed. This will immediately relieve the vena caval obstruction caused by the gravid uterus and improves survival rates for both mother and infant.

22. The reason for collapse was exsanguination from excessive blood loss. Cardiac electrical activity with no pulse is called 'pulseless electrical activity' (PEA). There is no need for adrenaline or cardiac shock since cardiac function and rhythm is normal. Due to exsanguination, cerebral perfusion is compromised and hence the loss of consciousness. Dobutamine is a sympathomimetic vasopressor drug which is of limited value in treating shock due to hypovolemia. It is more useful in toxin-induced hypotension from general

vasodilatation with normal blood volume, as in septicaemia. Atropine is a lifesaving parasympatholytic drug used to treat bradycardia in emergency situations, which is needed to maintain circulation to all vital organs. Calcium gluconate is reserved for cardiac arrest due to hypermagnesaemia (a potential risk in women treated with magnesium sulphate infusion as in severe pre-eclampsia).

23. This history is suggestive of concealed abruption and it is important to confirm foetal viability with a portable ultrasound scan. It will dictate mode of delivery while resuscitation is being carried out. Raised blood pressure may be seen in these patients but should not be treated with antihypertensive treatment.

24. If local anaesthetic toxicity is suspected (i.e. injected into a blood vessel), then stop injecting it immediately. The cardiac arrest team should be summoned. Treatment of cardiac arrest is with lipid emulsion (bolus injection of Intralipid 20%, followed by an intravenous infusion).

25. This woman is known to be asthmatic. It is likely that she had an acute anaphylaxis reaction, possibly to an insect bite. Basic life support should be provided and transferred to the hospital. The definitive treatment for anaphylaxis is 500 micrograms of 1:1,000 adrenaline intramuscularly (0.5 ml).

RCOG Green-top Guideline 56. Maternal collapse in pregnancy and the puerperium; 2021.

Answers for Questions 26–30

26. C; 27. B; 28. C; 29. A; 30. D

26. UKMEC category 3 includes conditions where the theoretical or proven risks generally outweigh the advantages of using the contraceptive method. COC users who smoke are at an increased risk of cardiovascular disease (in particular, myocardial infarction) compared to COC users who do not smoke. Any excess mortality associated with smoking is only apparent from age 35 years. The use of CHC use is therefore contraindicated from the age of 35 years (UKMEC 3 if below 15 cigarettes/day, or UKMEC 4 if more than 15 cigarettes/day). The cardiovascular disease risk associated with smoking decreases to that of a non-smoker within one to five years of stopping smoking.

27. UKMEC category 2 includes conditions where the advantages of using the contraceptive method generally outweigh the theoretical or proven risks. Valvular and congenital heart disease, even if associated with complications such as pulmonary hypertension, atrial fibrillation, or history of subacute bacterial endocarditis, are not a contraindication to intrauterine contraception (UKMEC 2). Prophylaxis against bacterial endocarditis is no longer indicated when inserting or removing a copper IUD or levonorgestrel IUS. Nulliparity is related to an increased risk of expulsion, but the benefits of using the method outweigh any disadvantages (UKMEC 2).

28. UKMEC category 3 includes conditions where the theoretical or proven risks generally outweigh the advantages of using the contraceptive method. Breast cancer is a hormonally sensitive tumour and therefore the prognosis of women with current or recent breast cancer may worsen if hormonal methods of contraception were used. This also applies to hormone receptor negative breast cancers. Current breast cancer is classified as UKMEC 4 (absolute contraindication), whereas a past history of breast cancer without any evidence of recurrence for five years ago is UKMEC 3.

29. UKMEC category 1 includes conditions where the advantages of using the contraceptive method generally outweigh the theoretical or proven risks. The use of a COC by women following evacuation of a molar pregnancy does not increase the risk of post-molar trophoblastic disease. Indeed there is some evidence that COC use by women in this

situation is associated with a more rapid regression in serum b-HCG levels than in women not using a COC. Advice should be sought from the specialist managing a woman's gestational trophoblastic disease as clinical guidelines vary in the UK.

30. UKMEC category 4 classifies conditions which represent an unacceptable risk if the contraceptive method is used. Multiple cardiovascular risk factors (such as older age, smoking, diabetes, hypertension, and obesity) may substantially increase the risk of cardiovascular disease and thus shift the woman into a higher UKMEC category. BMI 35 = UKMEC 3; smoking age <35 years = UKMEC 2; adequately controlled hypertension = UKMEC 3.

FSRH Guidelines & Statements—Faculty of Sexual and Reproductive Healthcare. Available at: https://www.fsrh.org/standards-and-guidance/fsrh-guidelines-and-statements/. (n.d.).

UK medical eligibility criteria (UKMEC) for contraceptive use | UKMEC 2016 (Amended September 2019).

Answers for Questions 31–36

31. K; 32. A; 33. C; 34. B; 35. D; 36. E

31. Stage 4B: Cancer has spread to distant organs or distant lymph nodes. The internal iliac nodes are not the first site of nodal spread (external iliac groin nodes) and are therefore classified as distant metastasis.

32. Stage 1A: This is defined as tumours that are 2 cm or less in their greatest diameter with no more than 1 mm of invasion into the underlying stroma.

33. Stage 2: The cancer has spread beyond the vulva or perineum to the anus or lower third of the vagina or urethra. It has not spread to lymph nodes or distant sites.

34. Stage 1B: These are stage 1 vulval cancers that have invaded deeper than 1 mm and/or are larger than 2 cm.

35. Stage 3A: Cancer is found in the vulva or perineum or both and may be growing into the anus, lower vagina, or lower urethra. It has either spread to a single nearby lymph node 5 mm or greater in size (3A1) or 1–2 lymph node metastasis/es under 5 mm in size (3A2).

36. Stage 3A2: The tumour may be any size with positive inguinofemoral lymph nodes with 1 or 2 lymph node metastasis below 5 mm in size. It has not spread to distant sites.

British Gynaecological Cancer Society/RCOG Guideline. Guidelines for the Diagnosis and Management of Vulval Carcinoma; 2014.

Answers for Questions 37–42

37. K; 38. H; 39. J; 40. A; 41. K; 42. C

37. Tibolone is an effective oral form of HRT that has combined oestrogenic, androgenic, and progestogenic effects. It must be given to women who are confirmed as being postmenopausal. It has been demonstrated in randomized controlled studies not to stimulate fibroid growth.

38. The options for the management of these women are limited. They cannot take HRT as they are likely to have had oestrogen-sensitive tumours. SSRIs in a limited number of well-controlled studies have shown short-term relief from vasomotor symptoms in about 50% of women.

39. HSDD in hysterectomized women who are taking oral oestrogen is a licensed indication for transdermal testosterone replacement.

40. A history of breast cancer would preclude HRT. Non-hormonal treatment such as alendronic acid should be considered.

41. Long-term treatment with LHRH-A will lead to ovarian suppression; thus oestrogen-deficiency symptoms such as hot flushes, osteopenia, and eventually osteoporosis are seen. Tibolone as an add-back therapy to HRT has a good safety record.

42. Local oestrogen treatment should be considered initially.

Burbos N, Morris E. Menopausal symptoms. BMJ Clinical Evidence; 2011.

Morris EP, Rymer J, Robinson J, Fogelman I. Efficacy of tibolone as 'add-back therapy' in conjunction with a gonadotropin-releasing hormone analogue in the treatment of uterine fibroids. *Fertil Steril* 2008;89(2):421–8.

Answers for Questions 43–47

43. B; 44. G; 45. C; 46. A; 47. I

43. It is a process to ensure that evidence-based practice forms the basis of clinical decision making. So the best evidence is available from the literature to provide the most effective, clinically relevant, and value-for-money care.

44. Under new commissioning arrangements in England and Wales, opinions are sought from the patients (user groups) and the public representatives to design local services which meet their aspirations. Patient involvement is important as their own experience of service use can define a patient-focused and user-friendly care pathway.

45. Clinical governance has been described as a framework for the continued improvement of patient care by minimizing clinical risks. This is an integrated approach to quality improvement throughout the whole organization. There is a proactive approach to reporting, dealing with, and learning from untoward incidents. Poor clinical performance is recognized, thus preventing potential harm to patients and staff.

46. Clinical audit is a systematic and critical analysis of the quality of clinical care, including the procedures used for diagnosis, treatment, use of resources, and the resulting outcome for the patient. Clinical audit seeks to improve the quality and outcome of patient care through continually examining and modifying practice according to standards set on the basis of the best available evidence.

47. A clinical risk is defined as 'a clinical error to be at variance from intended treatment, care, therapeutic intervention or a diagnostic result: thus there may be an untoward outcome or not'. Risk management is a strategy to develop good practice and reduce the occurrence of harmful or adverse incidents.

Healthcare Quality Improvement Partnership. Clinical audit: a guide for NHS boards and partners; March 2021.

Healthcare Quality Improvement Partnership. A guide to quality improvement tools; January 2021.

Answers for Questions 48–50

48. H; 49. E; 50. M

48. As this is an elderly patient in poor health, intraurethral bulking agents offer the best hope of improvement associated with the lowest morbidity. In addition, NASHA/DX can be injected under local anaesthesia in an outpatient setting.

49. Although long-term data are awaited, botulinum A toxin has been associated with good success rates and is less invasive than both neuromodulation and augmentation cystoplasty.

50. Current evidence suggests that TVT is the most appropriate procedure with the most complete outcome data, with the exception of colposuspension. TVT is less invasive than colposuspension. TOT could also be considered, but long-term data are lacking.

NICE Guideline 171. Urinary incontinence and pelvic organ prolapse in women: management; 2013.

paper

3

QUESTIONS

Single Best Answers

1. **A 24-year-old woman presents in clinic at 12 weeks gestation with monochorionic twins. Upon discussing the risks associated with monochorionic twins, she asks you how common twin-to-twin transfusion syndrome is. Which ONE of the following is the most appropriate answer?**
   A. 2%
   B. 5%
   C. 10%
   D. 20%
   E. 25%

2. **A GP refers a 58-year-old woman with a probable diagnosis of lichen sclerosis. Which ONE of the following is correct management?**
   A. A biopsy is required to confirm the diagnosis
   B. Topical steroids can be applied long term
   C. Topical treatment should include the vagina
   D. Treatment is required regardless of whether the woman has any symptoms
   E. Women should be seen every three months

3. **When presenting risk, the term 'very rare' is equivalent to:**
   A. 1 in 10,000
   B. 1 in 1,000
   C. A person in a large town
   D. A person in a small town
   E. A person in a village

4. **Of women who have recurrent pregnancy loss (i.e. three or more first-trimester miscarriages), what per cent will have anti-phospholipid antibodies?**
    A. 5%
    B. 15%
    C. 25%
    D. 30%
    E. 40%

5. **A 37-year-old primigravida woman presents at ten weeks gestation to the antenatal clinic. She has been referred because she has a known diagnosis of myasthenia gravis. Which ONE of the following is the most appropriate treatment?**
    A. Baclofen
    B. Beta-interferon
    C. Gabapentin
    D. Isoniazid
    E. Pyridostigmine

6. **At the gynaecology oncology multidisciplinary team meeting, a management plan is discussed for a 37-year-old woman diagnosed with breast cancer in pregnancy. She was diagnosed at nine weeks gestation with a tumour 2 cm in size. Which ONE of the following is the most appropriate treatment?**
    A. Surgical excision and chemotherapy as soon as possible, within the first trimester
    B. Surgical excision as soon as possible
    C. Surgical excision as soon as possible but administer chemotherapy in the second trimester
    D. Surgical excision as soon as possible, administering chemotherapy six weeks postoperatively
    E. Surgical excision in the second trimester

7. **You are asked to review the blood results of a 32-year-old woman at 28 weeks gestation in her second pregnancy. Which ONE of the following antibodies has significant risk of causing foetal anaemia at low titres?**
    A. Anti-C
    B. Anti-Duffy
    C. Anti-E
    D. Anti-Kell
    E. Anti-S

8. A 35-year-old woman is referred to see you with a 14-month history of secondary amenorrhoea. Which **ONE** of the following conditions is most commonly associated with premature ovarian failure?

    A. Hepatitis B
    B. Hypothyroidism
    C. Insulin-dependent diabetes mellitus
    D. Myasthenia gravis
    E. Rheumatoid arthritis

9. You are asked to review a 35-year-old woman in her first pregnancy at six weeks gestation. She has had a kidney transplant five years ago. Which **ONE** of the following is the complication most commonly seen in pregnant transplant recipients?

    A. Ectopic pregnancy
    B. Miscarriage
    C. Neonatal jaundice
    D. Oligohydramnios
    E. Placental abruption

10. You are discussing the complications associated with laparoscopic ovarian cystectomy. Which **ONE** of the following is associated with chemical peritonitis?

    A. Recurrence of an ovarian cyst
    B. Spillage of a cystadenoma
    C. Spillage of a dermoid cyst
    D. Spillage of an endometrioma
    E. Trocar site hernia

11. You are asked to review a woman who has sustained a vaginal tear following a normal delivery. On examination, you note that both the internal and external anal sphincters are torn; the anal epithelium remains intact. How would you classify this perineal tear?

    A. 3a tear
    B. 3b tear
    C. 3c tear
    D. Fourth-degree tear
    E. Deep

12. You review the ultrasound report of a 55-year-old woman with postmenopausal bleeding. At what endometrial thickness would you consider a pipelle biopsy?

    A. 3 mm
    B. 4 mm
    C. 5 mm
    D. 7 mm
    E. 9 mm

13. A 25-year-old woman presents in her second pregnancy at eight weeks gestation. She has previously had a painless preterm delivery at 26 weeks gestation, with no cause found. Which ONE of the following is correct?

A. Cerclage is recommended for funnelling of the cervix without cervical shortening

B. The insertion of a cerclage should be considered in women who have an incidentally identified short cervix of 25 mm length or less, regardless of their parity

C. PPROM is not a contraindication to cervical cerclage

D. Prophylactic cervical cerclage is recommended in women with a history of previous cervical cone biopsy

E. Transabdominal cerclage can be performed preconceptually or in early pregnancy

14. A 69-year-old woman presents with increasing irritation on her left labia. Which ONE of the following is true regarding management?

A. A biopsy should be taken immediately

B. A biopsy should be taken in three months if symptoms persist

C. Beta-interferon should be prescribed for treatment

D. Treatment is initially imiquimod

E. Treatment is initially topical Dermovate

15. A 32-year-old primigravid woman is referred to your antenatal clinic with a diagnosis of cytomegalovirus (CMV) infection. Which ONE of the following is true regarding CMV in pregnancy?

A. It can cause cataracts in the baby

B. It does not increase the risk of miscarriage

C. It is the most common viral infection transmitted to the foetus during labour

D. Treatment is by oral or parenteral pyrimethamine

E. Worldwide 5% of foetuses are affected

16. A couple with a three-year history of infertility of unknown aetiology come to see you regarding IVF. Which ONE of the following is correct?

A. Consider double embryo transfer in women aged 40 and over, even in the presence of top-quality embryo

B. In women aged 40–42 years who have not conceived after two years of regular unprotected intercourse or 12 cycles of artificial insemination, one full cycle of IVF with or without ICSI should be considered, irrespective of whether they have had IVF treatment previously

C. In women less than 40 years of age who have not conceived after two years of regular unprotected intercourse or 12 cycles of artificial insemination, two full cycles of IVF should be offered, with or without ICSI

D. Natural cycle IVF treatment and the use of ovarian stimulation are both recommended as part of IVF treatment

E. Ultrasound monitoring of the ovarian response is an integral part of the IVF treatment cycle

17. **You are taking over as the registrar on call for the labour ward. The midwife in charge tells you that all of the rooms are full and that she is short-staffed. Which ONE of the following patients would you see first?**

   A. A 19-year-old postnatal patient on serenity suite (24 weeks intrauterine foetal death following prolonged pre-labour rupture of membranes), feeling unwell with pyrexia and tachycardia; you note she has two red scores on the MEOWS chart with reduced urinary output

   B. A 26-year-old woman with breech presentation (planned elective caesarean section at 39 weeks) admitted with spontaneous rupture of membranes at 38 weeks gestation

   C. A 27-year-old primiparous woman in labour, whose cervical dilatation has remained unchanged at 4 cm after four hours of syntocinon augmentation

   D. A suspicious CTG in a 34-year-old multiparous woman who has been actively pushing for 30 minutes

   E. A third-degree tear waiting to be sutured, having given birth two hours ago; bleeding is minimal

18. **A 25-year-old woman presents with a history of vaginal bleeding and pelvic cramps. She is eight weeks pregnant. Which ONE of the following is consistent with the ultrasound diagnosis of a miscarriage?**

   A. Crown rump length of 5 mm with an absent foetal heartbeat

   B. Crown rump length of 7 mm with an absent foetal heartbeat

   C. Mean gestational sac diameter of 8 mm with no growth over five days

   D. Mean gestational sac diameter of 20 mm with no foetal pole

   E. The presence of a yolk sac and an amniotic sac with an embryonic pole with no cardiac activity

19. **A 24-year-old woman presents at 27 weeks gestation with lower abdominal pain. She has palpable tightening every ten minutes. Which ONE of the following groups of drugs should be prescribed first-line for tocolysis?**

   A. Beta-antagonists

   B. Calcium channel blockers

   C. Magnesium sulphate

   D. Nitric oxide donors

   E. Oxytocin receptor agonists

20. **A 34-year-old woman presents with severe hyperemesis gravidarum and is admitted for rehydration and intravenous anti-emetic therapy. An ultrasound shows features suggestive of a 'snowstorm' in-utero. Which ONE of the following is correct in relation to the most likely diagnosis?**
    A. Dietary factors, such as poor intake of vitamin A, are linked to complete molar pregnancies
    B. Pregnancy should be avoided for six months following completion of chemotherapy treatment
    C. Surgical evacuation is recommended when ultrasound has shown a twin pregnancy consisting of a molar pregnancy and viable foetus
    D. There is a 0.5% chance of requiring chemotherapy with a complete molar pregnancy
    E. Triploidy is associated with a complete molar pregnancy

21. **A 24-year-old woman requests the combined oral contraceptive pill (COCP) for contraception. With which ONE of the following conditions is the COCP safe to prescribe?**
    A. Benign liver tumours
    B. BMI ≥ 40 kg/m^2
    C. Family history of thromboembolism
    D. Previous history of gestational trophoblastic neoplasia with currently high HCG
    E. Valvular heart disease complicated by atrial fibrillation

22. **A 37-year-old woman in her second pregnancy has come to see you following the ultrasound finding of a myelomeningocele. Which ONE of the following is true?**
    A. A banana-shaped cerebellum is seen on ultrasound scan in more than 99% of cases
    B. Hydrocephalus is present in <50% of cases
    C. Most myelomeningoceles originate at the level of cervical and thoracic spine
    D. Only the meninges protrude through the spine and look like a sac on ultrasound scan
    E. A strawberry-shaped skull is common on ultrasound scan

23. **A 42-year-old HIV-positive woman attends following the finding of HR HPV and CIN 1 on her cytology report. Which ONE of the following statements is correct?**
    A. All HIV-positive women should attend for annual cytology with an initial colposcopy
    B. CIN 1 affects the superficial third of the epithelial layer
    C. CIN 1 is an indication for cold coagulation or laser ablation
    D. CIN 1 is an indication for large loop excision of the transformation zone (LLETZ)
    E. HIV-positive women should attend for annual colposcopy

24. **The last MBRRACE-UK Confidential Enquiry was recently published in the UK. Which ONE of the following statements is true of maternal mortality?**
    A. Globally, there is still a worrying increase in the number of maternal deaths
    B. In the last MBRRACE-UK Confidential Enquiry, the commonest cause of direct deaths in the UK was due to thrombosis and thromboembolism
    C. In the UK, the gap in the maternal mortality rates between the social classes is now reducing
    D. Maternal mortality rate in the UK is defined as the number of direct and indirect deaths per 100,000 live births
    E. The Millennium Development Goal 5 is to improve women's health by funding developing countries to build more maternity units

25. **You perform a transvaginal ultrasound scan on a 46-year-old woman who has a unilateral ovarian cyst. Which ONE of the following is a suspicious feature?**
    A. An ovarian cyst over 10 cm in maximal diameter
    B. The presence of acoustic shadowing in a 5 cm ovarian cyst
    C. The presence of a papillary structure in a 7 cm ovarian cyst
    D. A regular multilocular 8 cm cyst
    E. A smooth multilocular 3 cm cyst with calcified areas

26. **A 42-year-old woman complains of increasing perineal pain six hours following a ventouse delivery and episiotomy. On examination, she is pale and tachycardic. Perineal inspection reveals a right-sided tense 4 cm vulval haematoma. In vulval hematoma, the extension of bleeding in the anterior triangle is limited by which of the following?**
    A. Anal fascia
    B. Camper's fascia
    C. Colles' fascia
    D. Denonvilliers' fascia
    E. Scarpa's fascia

27. **A 25-year-old HIV-positive woman presents in her first pregnancy. Which ONE of the following is true regarding treatment?**
    A. All women should have commenced combined antiretroviral therapy by week 24 of pregnancy
    B. For women who do not require HIV treatment for their own health, either zidovudine monotherapy or highly active antiretroviral therapy (HAART) should be initiated by 24 weeks
    C. Pregnant HIV-positive women should take antiretroviral therapy if CD4 count is below 100 cells/mcL
    D. When a woman is asymptomatic, with a high CD4 + count and low viral load, treatment should be started at the end of the second trimester of pregnancy
    E. With treatment, HIV is vertically transmitted in approximately 25% of cases

28. **A 25-year-old woman undergoes an emergency caesarean section (CS) at full dilatation, following a failed instrumental delivery. Regarding CS at full dilatation, which ONE of the following is correct?**
    A. CS at full dilatation is associated with almost double the risk of intraoperative trauma
    B. Frequency of constipation is higher at one year with CS at full dilatation
    C. Increased maternal BMI increases the risk of CS at full dilatation
    D. Risk of wound infection is higher with a CS at full dilatation than with operative delivery
    E. Women undergoing an operative vaginal delivery are less likely to report difficulty in conceiving and more likely to have a further pregnancy than those who undergo a CS

29. **Your junior trainee sees a 39-year-old primigravid woman who is eight weeks pregnant and demanding aspirin therapy. Which ONE of the following is an indication to prescribe low-dose aspirin?**
    A. BMI greater than 35 kg/m² at booking
    B. Multiple pregnancy
    C. Pregnancy interval over ten years
    D. Primigravida and maternal age 39
    E. Primigravida and maternal age 42

30. **A 24-year-old woman in her second pregnancy is diagnosed with placenta praevia accreta, following an open myomectomy and elective caesarean section. Which ONE of the following is correct management?**
    A. Grey-scale ultrasound complemented by colour Doppler and three-dimensional power Doppler remains the imaging modality of choice with sensitivity up to 80% and specificity up to 75%
    B. Magnetic resonance imaging should be performed first-line to diagnose the morbidly adherent placenta
    C. Methotrexate should be administered to reduce the risk of bleeding in women with retained placenta accreta following delivery
    D. Prophylactic placement of arterial catheters at the time of delivery should be performed
    E. Regional anaesthesia is not contraindicated for delivery for placenta praevia or suspected placenta accreta

31. **The NHS Fetal Anomaly Screening Programme (FASP) routinely screens for the following conditions, except for which ONE of the following?**
    A. Anencephaly
    B. Bilateral renal agenesis
    C. Diaphragmatic hernia
    D. Gastroschisis
    E. Phaeochromocytoma

32. **Which ONE of the following genetic disorders is correctly linked to its transmission type?**
    A. Cystic fibrosis is transmitted as an autosomal recessive disease
    B. Factor VII deficiency is transmitted as an autosomal dominant disease
    C. Huntington's disease is transmitted as a single gene mutation
    D. Marfan's syndrome transmission is a sex-linked disease
    E. Neurofibromatosis type 1 is transmitted as an autosomal recessive disease

33. **A 24-year-old woman attends your clinic for emergency contraception after two episodes of unprotected sexual intercourse over the last 24 hours. She is currently on treatment for tuberculosis. Which ONE of the following is the most appropriate contraceptive to prescribe her?**
    A. Copper intrauterine device
    B. Implanon
    C. Levonorgestrel
    D. Mirena intrauterine system
    E. Ulipristal acetate

34. **A 24-year-old woman presenting with a history of menorrhagia is found to have a 4 cm simple left ovarian cyst. Which ONE of the following is the most appropriate management?**
    A. Obtain consent for laparoscopic left ovarian aspiration
    B. Obtain consent for laparoscopic left ovarian cystectomy
    C. Repeat the ultrasound in four weeks
    D. Request serum CA125
    E. Routine follow-up is not required and the patient should be reassured

35. **A 60-year-old woman presents with a history of recurrent vaginal bleeding. Which ONE of the following is a risk factor for endometrial cancer?**
    A. Cigarette smoking
    B. Diabetes
    C. Multiparity
    D. Obesity
    E. Ovarian endometrioma

36. **A 45-year-old woman has urodynamic stress incontinence and is keen to avoid surgery. Which ONE of the following non-surgical treatment options is most likely to improve her symptoms?**
    A. Alteration of fluid management
    B. Constipation relief
    C. Smoking cessation
    D. Specialist physiotherapy
    E. Vaginal oestrogens

37. **A 23-year-old woman presents with a two-day history of no foetal movements at 28 weeks gestation. Ultrasound scan confirms an intrauterine death. You are asked to prescribe misoprostol. What regimen will you prescribe?**

A. 50 µg per vagina four hourly

B. 50 µg orally six hourly

C. 100 µg orally four hourly

D. 100 µg per vagina six hourly

E. 200 µg per vagina six hourly

38. **A 36-year-old woman presents to the outpatient hysteroscopy clinic with heavy menstrual bleeding for the last six months with symptomatic anaemia. She has not completed her family. A preliminary ultrasound showed a bulky uterus with a 3 cm hypoechoic mass, deviating from the endometrial echo suggesting a fibroid. Which ONE of the following is the most appropriate management plan?**

A. Hysterectomy with preservation of the ovaries

B. Hysteroscopic resection of submucous fibroid

C. Mirena intrauterine system

D. Tranexamic acid

E. Uterine artery embolization

39. **Male factor infertility is noted in one-third of the fertility cases. Which ONE of the following is true regarding male factor infertility?**

A. According to WHO a semen analysis, a result with a sperm count of 15 million per ml, motility of 60%, and morphology of 4% is normal

B. Cervical mucous post-coital testing is recommended to improve the pregnancy rate

C. If the result of the first semen analysis is suboptimal, a repeat test is recommended after three months with encouragement for healthy lifestyle changes

D. Mild male factor infertility is defined as two or more semen analyses with one or more variables below the 10th centile

E. Screening for anti-sperm antibodies should be offered

40. **A 23-year-old primiparous woman is diagnosed to have a miscarriage at eight weeks gestation. Which ONE of the following is correct regarding management?**

A. Anti-D should be given to all non-sensitized Rhesus-negative women who miscarry after eight weeks gestation

B. Conservative management has an average success rate of 80%

C. Infection rate is similar regardless of whether medical, surgical, or expectant management is undertaken

D. Mifepristone increases the efficacy of misoprostol in the management of miscarriage

E. The number of days of bleeding is less with surgical treatment than expectant management

41. **A 32-year-old woman comes in with vaginal bleeding. She is 12 weeks pregnant and noted to be Rhesus status negative. Which ONE of the following is true regarding anti-D prophylaxis in pregnancy?**

    A. Anti-D immunoglobulin should be administered to all Rhesus-negative women who attend with a threatened miscarriage at 11 + 6 weeks

    B. Anti-D immunoglobulin should be administered at monthly intervals in Rhesus-negative women with persistent vaginal bleeding after 20 completed weeks of pregnancy

    C. Anti-D immunoglobulin should ideally be administered in the gluteus muscle

    D. Over 50% of significant (>4 ml) fetomaternal haemorrhages will occur during normal vaginal delivery

    E. Routine testing to quantify the size of the fetomaternal haemorrhage is not recommended in the UK

42. **You are asked for advice on a 15-year-old girl who has been raped. She has not washed since the incident. During the course of the forensic medical examination, a range of forensic samples are taken. Which ONE of the following is correct?**

    A. The time limit for detection of body fluids in the vagina following digital penetration is 12 hours

    B. The time limit for detection of body fluids, cellular material, or lubricants on the skin is 24 hours

    C. The time limit for detection of semen in the mouth is 24 hours following oral penetration

    D. The time limit for detection of semen in the rectum following anal penetration is 48 hours

    E. The time limit for detection of semen in the vagina following vaginal penetration in a post-pubertal female is 120 hours (five days)

43. **A 36-year-old woman in her first pregnancy has been referred to see you at 39 weeks gestation. She is upset on finding out that her baby is in breech presentation. What is the incidence of spontaneous version from breech to cephalic presentation in nulliparous women after 36 weeks?**

    A. 2%

    B. 4%

    C. 6%

    D. 8%

    E. 10%

44. **A 34-year-old primigravid woman presents in labour, having been pushing for 75 minutes. You are asked to review whether she is suitable for an operative vaginal delivery. Which ONE of the following is correct?**

A. Epidural with oxytocin in the second stage of labour increases the incidence of non-rotational forceps delivery in primiparous women

B. Foetal alloimmune thrombocytopenia is a relative contraindication to operative vaginal delivery

C. Instrumental delivery is contraindicated if any part of the foetal head is palpable abdominally

D. Maternal BMI over 30 is not associated with a higher rate of failed instrumental delivery, until BMI is over 40

E. Ventouse delivery is safe beyond 35 weeks of gestation

45. **A 33-year-old woman is diagnosed to have severe ovarian hyperstimulation syndrome (OHSS). Which ONE of the following is the most appropriate management?**

A. Diuretics should be used in women with oliguria

B. Multidisciplinary assistance is needed when initial crystalloid and colloid therapy fails, leading to persistent haemoconcentration and dehydration

C. Paracentesis should not be considered as it might worsen her symptoms

D. Surgery is recommended in women who do not respond to conservative treatment to reduce ovarian size

E. Women should be reassured that pregnancy may continue normally despite OHSS, and there is evidence of an increased risk of congenital abnormalities

46. **A 42-year-old woman is asked to see you in the antenatal clinic. She has had previous caesarean section and is keen to try for a vaginal delivery. Which ONE of the following factors decreases the likelihood of a successful vaginal birth after caesarean section (VBAC)?**

A. Epidural labour analgesia

B. Previous caesarean section for dystocia

C. Previous caesarean section for foetal distress

D. Previous caesarean section for foetal malpresentation

E. VBAC at or after 41 weeks of gestation

47. **A 24-year-old woman attends labour ward at 35 weeks' gestation with a history of no foetal movements and leaking clear fluid vaginally continuously over the last four hours. Ultrasound confirms oligohydramnios and no foetal heartbeat. She is fit and well, other than a diagnosis of group B Streptococcus noted at 28 weeks gestation, and her observations are normal. Which ONE of the following is your next step for management?**

A. Administer intravenous antibiotics

B. Administer oral misoprostol

C. Expectant management

D. Insert a transcervical balloon catheter

E. A single dose of mifepristone to reduce the duration of labour

48. **You are asked to review a 68-year-old woman presenting with a six-month history of increasing vulval pruritus and a small area of irregularity on her left labial fold, suggestive of vulvar intraepithelial neoplasia (VIN). Which ONE of the following is correct?**
    A. 1% of women with VIN have intraepithelial neoplasia at other lower genital tract sites
    B. 10% of women with VIN have intraepithelial neoplasia at other lower genital tract sites
    C. The incidence of VIN 3 is 1 in 10,000
    D. Risk factors include immunosuppression
    E. Treatment is initially topical Dermovate

49. **A 48-year-old woman presents with heavy menstrual bleeding and urinary frequency. An ultrasound shows a 7 cm anterior wall submucosal fibroid. Regarding treatment, which ONE of the following is correct?**
    A. Endometrial ablation reduces the size of fibroid
    B. High-dose oral progestogen may decrease the size of fibroid
    C. Hysterectomy is a definitive cure for heavy menstrual bleeding associated with fibroid
    D. A levonorgestrel-containing intrauterine device does not decrease size of fibroid
    E. Tranexamic acid may decrease the size of fibroid

50. **A 30-year-old woman comes to see you with urinary incontinence three months after a normal delivery. Regarding urinary symptoms, which ONE of the following indicate abnormal urine storage?**
    A. Frequency and nocturia
    B. Hesitancy and poor stream
    C. Post-micturition dribble and incomplete emptying
    D. Straining to void and painful bladder
    E. Urgency and dysuria

Extended Matching Questions

Options for Questions 1–5

For each of the case histories described, choose the single most likely cause of breathlessness from the list provided. Each option may be used once, more than once, or not at all.

- A. Amniotic fluid embolism
- B. Anaemia
- C. Diabetic ketoacidosis
- D. Hyperventilation
- E. Hypoglycaemia
- F. Myocardial infarction
- G. Peripartum cardiomyopathy
- H. Physiological
- I. Pneumonia
- J. Pneumothorax
- K. Pulmonary embolism
- L. Status asthmaticus

1. A fit 28-year-old woman develops a sudden onset of chest pain during the active second stage. The pain worsened after delivery and was associated with a severe onset of breathlessness. There was reduced air entry on one side of the chest and percussion of the same side revealed a hyper-resonant note.

2. A slim 41-year-old multiparous woman developed breathlessness on the 10th day following delivery and self-referred herself to the emergency department. She is tachycardic, and X-ray showed evidence of pulmonary oedema. Her CTPA was negative for pulmonary embolus.

3. A 19-year-old primigravid woman presents to obstetric triage with breathlessness associated with paraesthesia of hands. Her arterial blood gas shows a normal pO_2, but slightly reduced pCO_2.

4. A 22-year-old insulin-dependent diabetic presents for assessment at 14 weeks gestation in her first pregnancy. Blood sugars have previously been well-controlled on insulin and she has just been started on antibiotics for a urinary tract infection. She has been feeling increasingly confused and unwell over the preceding three hours with deep and laboured breathing. She has vomited twice and appears clinically dehydrated.

5. A 40-year-old woman on the gynaecology ward is being managed for moderate OHSS. She is complaining of new onset shortness of breath at rest, although her abdominal girth has reduced and blood investigations remain normal.

Options for Questions 6–10

For each of the following clinical scenarios, select the most appropriate form of thromboprophylaxis. Each option may be used once, more than once, or not at all.

- A. High-dose LMWH antenatally and six weeks postnatally
- B. High-dose LMWH antenatally and six weeks postnatally followed by long-term anticoagulation
- C. High-dose LMWH one week postnatally
- D. High-dose LMWH six weeks postnatally
- E. Low-dose aspirin and low-dose LMWH

F. Low-dose aspirin antenatally and six weeks postnatally

G. Low-dose aspirin six weeks postnatally

H. Prophylactic dose LMWH antenatally and six weeks postnatally

I. Prophylactic dose LMWH for ten days postnatally

J. Prophylactic dose LMWH six weeks postnatally

K. Thromboprophylactic stockings one week postnatally

L. No thromboprophylaxis required

6. A 36-year-old primiparous woman who is known to be heterozygous for factor V Leiden. She has no other risk factors and has just delivered her second baby.

7. A 24-year-old primiparous woman with no history of thromboembolism but is known to be homozygous for factor V Leiden. She has no other risk factors.

8. A 28-year-old multiparous woman who has a BMI 42 kg/m^2 but otherwise has no other risk factors.

9. A 32-year-old multiparous woman who had a deep vein thrombosis in her last pregnancy but no other risk factors.

10. A 27-year-old primiparous woman who is known to have antiphospholipid syndrome and a previous pulmonary embolism.

Options for Questions 11–15

The following clinical scenarios describe situations in which the use of one or more contraceptive methods is not advisable. For each scenario, decide which contraceptive method or methods should be avoided from the list of available options; assume that there are no other factors that influence contraceptive suitability. Each option may be used once, more than once, or not at all.

A. All hormonal contraceptive methods, excluding the levonorgestrel-containing intrauterine system (IUS)

B. All hormonal contraceptive methods, including the levonorgestrel-containing IUS

C. Combined hormonal contraception (CHC), combined oral contraceptive pill (COCP), combined vaginal ring (CVR), combined transdermal patch (CTP)

D. CHC and progestogen-only injectables (Depo-Provera®)

E. Copper-containing intrauterine contraceptive device (IUD)

F. Copper-containing intrauterine contraceptive device (IUD) and progestogen-only pill (POP)

G. Levonorgestrel-containing IUS

H. Levonorgestrel-containing IUS and copper-containing intrauterine contraceptive device (IUD)

I. Progestogen-only implants

J. Progestogen-only injectables (Depo-Provera®)

K. Progestogen-only pill (POP)

L. Progestogen-only pill (POP) and progestogen-only implants

M. All of the above

N. None of the above

11. A 30-year-old nulliparous woman with systemic lupus erythematosus (SLE) with positive or unknown antiphospholipid antibodies.

12. A 26-year-old woman with chronic viral hepatitis with normal liver function.

13. A 33-year-old woman with a family history of venous thromboembolism (VTE) in a first-degree relative under the age of 45 years. Patient has normal thrombophilia screen.

14. A 27-year-old nulliparous woman with a history of an ectopic pregnancy managed by salpingectomy. She has been found to have two submucosal fibroids which are distorting the uterine cavity.

15. A 22-year-old woman with insulin-dependent diabetes with neuropathy and microvascular disease.

Options for Questions 16–20

For each of the following cases, choose the correct cervical cancer FIGO stage. Each option may be used once, more than once, or not at all.

    A. Stage 1A1
    B. Stage 1A2
    C. Stage 1B1
    D. Stage 1B2
    E. Stage 2A1
    F. Stage 2A2
    G. Stage 2B
    H. Stage 3A
    I. Stage 3B
    J. Stage 4A
    K. Stage 4B
    L. More information needed in order to stage
    M. None of the above

16. A 42-year-old woman who is known to have squamous cell carcinoma of the cervix undergoes cystoscopy. A suspicious lesion is found and a biopsy from the bladder mucosa confirms spread. There are no other signs of metastases on subsequent examination and investigation.

17. A 30-year-old woman has CIN 3 which is confirmed following a LLETZ. The margins are clear.

18. A 56-year-old woman known to have squamous cell cervical carcinoma is found to have parametrial spread only without involvement of the pelvic sidewall and lower third of vagina on subsequent examination and investigations.

19. A 35-year-old woman undergoes a LLETZ for an abnormal smear. Histology confirms a microscopic invasive squamous cell carcinoma with a measured maximal stromal invasion of 2.0 mm in depth and extension of 5.5 mm. The margins are clear and there is no evidence of spread.

20. A 42-year-old woman has a clinically visible lesion on her cervix measuring 5.5 cm in maximum dimension which is subsequently proven to be a squamous cell carcinoma of the cervix on histology.

Options for Questions 21–25

For each of the following cases, choose the correct immediate management plan. Each option may be used once, more than once, or not at all.

    A. Antibiotics iv
    B. Arterial blood gas
    C. Blood transfusion
    D. Chest X-ray
    E. Colloid infusion iv
    F. Crystalloid infusion iv
    G. Dobutamine infusion

H. Emergency caesarean section

I. Exchange transfusion

J. Hysterectomy

K. ITU admission

L. Steroids im

M. Steroids iv

N. Uterine artery embolization

21. A 24-year-old woman at 26 weeks of pregnancy presents to the labour ward with a history of prolonged rupture of membranes. She is cold and clammy and, despite preliminary resuscitation, has a blood pressure of 70/40 mmHg. Her arterial blood gas shows pH 7.27; pO_2 7.6; pCO_2 5.4; lactate 6.7. What will be your next plan of management for her?

22. A 32-year-old woman with known sickle cell disease presents at 32 weeks of pregnancy with severe shortness of breath and chest pain. Her recent blood test shows a haemoglobin of 5.2 g/dl and a high reticulocyte count. What will be your next plan of management for her?

23. A 40-year-old woman, at term, is in labour with a history of 56 hours of prolonged rupture of membranes. She suddenly develops a temperature of 40°C and has rigors. What will be your next course of action?

24. A 28-year-old pregnant woman is now 30 weeks pregnant after having an emergency cerclage inserted at 20 weeks. The midwife calls you to review her because she has suddenly developed high-grade pyrexia, with a maternal and foetal tachycardia of 140 bpm and 180 bpm, respectively. Initial resuscitation has been completed. What will be your plan of management for her?

25. A 42-year-old postpartum woman is blue-lighted to the labour ward in septic and haemorrhagic shock. She had a normal delivery seven days ago and has now come in with high-grade pyrexia and having lost 3 litres of blood via vagina. Her blood pressure is 80/40 mmHg and heart rate 120 bpm. Arterial blood gas shows Hb 8.2 g/dl, lactate 4.5. What is your most appropriate immediate management?

Options for Questions 26–30

For each of the following clinical scenarios, choose the most appropriate response. Each option may be used once, more than once, or not at all.

A. Acute abdomen

B. Acute pyelonephritis

C. Breast abscess

D. Caesarean section wound infection

E. Cholecystitis

F. Cystitis

G. Group A Streptococcus septicaemia

H. Group B Streptococcus septicaemia

I. Infected episiotomy

J. Mastitis

K. Infected perineal tears

L. Pelvic sepsis

M. Venous thromboembolism

26. A 35-year-old woman underwent an emergency caesarean section after failure to progress. On the fifth day postoperatively, she complains of abdominal and pelvic pain. Her temperature

was 38.5°C and her abdomen is tender on palpation, more so on the right side. She is able to mobilize but bends forward when doing so.

27. A 30-year-old woman is admitted at 29 weeks with an intrauterine death. She delivers vaginally but 24 hours later starts to complain of fever and shortness of breath. Her respiratory rate is 20 breaths per minute and she is admitted to HDU.

28. A 34-year-old woman complains of difficulty passing urine and has a fever. She is day two following a forceps delivery for a prolonged second stage.

29. A 24-year-old woman underwent a normal vaginal delivery and is breastfeeding. On day six post-delivery, her district nurse notes that she is feverish (temperature 38.2°C), and is experiencing difficulty in passing urine. One of her breasts is tender and hot to touch.

30. A 39-year-old primiparous white woman with a BMI of 42 has a manual removal of placenta. On day five following the procedure she is seen in the acute medical unit complaining of right-sided abdominal pain and vomiting. On examination, there is tenderness in the upper abdomen.

Options for Questions 31–35

For each of the following scenarios, choose the correct terminology. Each option may be used once, more than once, or not at all.

- A. Autonomy
- B. Beneficence
- C. Bichard guidance
- D. Competency
- E. Confidentiality
- F. Disclosure
- G. Fraser guidelines
- H. Gillick competence
- I. Justice
- J. Non-maleficence
- K. Paternalism
- L. Refusal of consent

31. Physicians must act in the best interests of their patients.

32. The moral obligation to act on the basis of fair adjudication between competing claims.

33. The physician must 'do no harm' to patients.

34. A patient's right to privacy regarding their medical care.

35. The interference with or failure to respect affairs normally designated as matters within an individual's sphere of liberty for the sake of that individual.

Options for Questions 36–40

Select the most appropriate term for the type of study described. Each option may be used once, more than once, or not at all.

- A. Anonymized case reporting
- B. Case-controlled
- C. Clinical audit
- D. Cohort
- E. Crossover design
- F. Intention to treat

G. NHS safety alerts

H. Patient-related outcomes

I. Prospective

J. Quasi-randomized

K. Randomized controlled

L. Retrospective

36. A study to compare the care profile of patients who underwent hysterectomy either laparoscopically or by standard open approach in a tertiary centre by review of case notes.

37. A study to assess the outcomes of small-for-gestational-age neonates born in a district general hospital over two-year period, and to record their developmental milestones at one, two, and five years.

38. A study to assess which regimen would provide better glycaemic control in nulliparous pregnant patients diagnosed with gestational diabetes: for the first four weeks, one group of primiparous women are to be treated with metformin and insulin, the second group with metformin alone; in week five, the treatments are switched over.

39. A study to analyse maternal and foetal outcomes for caesarean sections performed at full cervical dilation in a tertiary level centre over the past two years.

40. The RCOG has published a new guideline on infertility. An auditable standard was identified to assess different techniques for the evaluation of tubal function among infertile women in this population.

Options for Questions 41–45

For each of the following clinical scenarios, choose the most appropriate next step from the list provided. Each option may be used once, more than once, or not at all.

A. Blastomere pre-implantation biopsy

B. Clomiphene

C. Cytogenetic studies

D. Donor insemination

E. Expectant treatment

F. Folic acid

G. GnRH analogues

H. ICSI

I. IUI

J. IVF

K. LH-timed intercourse

L. Ovarian biopsy

M. Pre-implantation embryo biopsy

N. Regular unprotected sexual intercourse

41. A 28-year-old woman with a history of five previous miscarriages under ten weeks of gestation presents with heavy vaginal bleeding at nine weeks of gestation.

42. A 32-year-old woman with primary infertility for 17 months. Her anti-Müllerian hormone level is 2.

43. A 30-year-old woman with a known autosomal recessive single gene disorder who has been trying to conceive for eight months. She is timing intercourse with her partner with ovulation and has a regular menstrual cycle.

44. A 30-year-old nulliparous woman who is in a same-sex relationship. Neither partner has been pregnant before.

45. A 35-year-old nulliparous diabetic woman who is well-controlled on insulin and is considering infertility treatment.

Options for Questions 46–50

For each of the following clinical scenarios, choose the most appropriate next step from the list provided. Each option may be used once, more than once, or not at all.

    A. Chromosomal analysis of both partners
    B. Chromosomal analysis of female partner
    C. Factor V Leiden testing
    D. Free androgen index
    E. Hysteroscopy
    F. Laparoscopy
    G. MRI of genitourinary system
    H. Natural killer cell antibodies screening
    I. Progesterone level estimation
    J. Prophylactic cervical cerclage
    K. Reassurance
    L. Thrombophilia screening
    M. Torch screen
    N. Ultrasound scan for cervical length during pregnancy
    O. Weight loss

46. A 25-year-old nulliparous woman with a BMI of 28, with normal ovulatory cycles, has had two confirmed pregnancy losses at 8–9 weeks gestation.

47. A 38-year-old nulliparous woman with a BMI of 40 presents with an irregular menstrual cycle. She has had one pregnancy loss at ten weeks gestation at the age of 36.

48. A 21-year-old woman with a regular menstrual cycle is referred following her fourth first-trimester miscarriage. Her BMI is 25 and a laparoscopy for tubal patency was reported as normal.

49. A 32-year-old woman with a history of painless rupture of membranes at 22 weeks in two pregnancies, leading to a pregnancy loss a few weeks later.

50. A 34-year-old woman with a history of three pregnancy losses between eight and nine weeks. Following her third loss, products of conception were sent for cytogenetic studies suggesting some chromosomal abnormality.

paper
3

Single Best Answers

1. C. 10%

TTTS is seen in 10–15% of all monochorionic pregnancies and is associated with multiple placental vascular anastomoses between the foetal circulations. Without treatment, it is associated with an 80–100% mortality rate; 15–50% risk of disability is seen among those who survive.

Morris RK, Chan BC, Kilby M. Advances in fetal therapy. *TOG* 2010;12:94–102.

2. B. Topical steroids can be applied long term

Histological diagnosis is reserved for diagnostically difficult cases or those which are resistant to treatment. The vagina and cervix are generally not affected and treatment is required only if symptoms occur. The frequency of follow-up is variable, but bleeding and ulceration should be reported. Vulval steroids can be applied safely long term.

BSVVD. Standards of Care for patients with vulval conditions; 2022.

Kingston A. The postmenopausal vulva. *TOG* 2012;11(4):252–9.

3. C. A person in a large town.

The RCOG Clinical Governance Advice, 'Presenting information on risk', defines the following terms:

Very common: 1 in 1 to 1 in 10 (a person in the family)

Common: 1 in 10 to 1 in 100 (a person in the street)

Uncommon: 1 in 100 to 1 in 1,000 (a person in a village)

Rare: 1 in 1,000 to 1 in 10,000 (a person in a small town)

Very rare: Less than 1 in 10,000 (a person in a large town)

RCOG Clinical Governance Advice 1. Presenting information on risk; 2008.

Adapted by permission from BMJ Publishing Group Limited. *The BMJ*, Calman KC and Royston G, 'Personal paper: Risk language and dialects', 315, p. 939, copyright 1997, with permission from BMJ Publishing Group Ltd.

4. B. 15%

In women with recurrent pregnancy loss, 10–20% have detectable antiphospholipid antibodies. If left untreated, the risk of a further pregnancy loss can be up to 90%.

Myers B, Pavord S. Diagnosis and management of antiphospholipid syndrome in pregnancy. *TOG* 2011;13:15–21.

5. E. Pyridostigmine

Myasthenia gravis is a rare autoimmune condition caused by antibodies against the nicotinic acetylcholine receptors. It is more commonly seen in women, and 40% have an exacerbation in pregnancy. Pyridostigmine is a long-acting anticholinesterase drug used to treat myasthenia gravis. Other medications which may also be considered include corticosteroids, azathioprine, and plasmaphoresis.

Nelson-Piercy C. *Obstetric medicine*, 6th ed. Boca Raton: CRC Press; 2020.

6. C. Surgical excision as soon as possible but administer chemotherapy in the second trimester

Breast surgery can be performed safely at any gestation of pregnancy with little risk to the foetus. However, the timing of chemotherapy is crucial. A delay in chemotherapy of over three weeks following surgery is thought to have a significant impact on the prognosis compared with early commencement of chemotherapy. Chemotherapy is safe in the second and third trimester. It should be avoided in the first trimester due to the risk of foetal malformation and miscarriage.

Padmagirison R, Gajjar K, Spencer C. Management of breast cancer during pregnancy. *TOG* 2010;12:186–92.

RCOG Green-top Guideline 12. Pregnancy and breast cancer; 2011.

7. D. Anti-Kell

Red cell alloimmunization rarely affects a first pregnancy, whilst platelet antigen alloimmunization can affect a first pregnancy. Antibodies which have a significant risk of causing foetal anaemia include anti-C, anti-D, and anti-Kell. For anti-K antibodies, referral should take place once detected as severe foetal anaemia can occur even with low titres.

Gajjar K, Spencer C. Diagnosis and management of non-anti-D red cell antibodies in pregnancy. *TOG* 2009;11:89–95.

RCOG Green-top Guidelines 65. The management of women with red cell antibodies during pregnancy; 2014.

8. B. Hypothyroidism

13.8% of women with premature ovarian failure have associated hypothyroidism, whilst 1.7% have insulin-dependent diabetes mellitus. The cause of premature ovarian failure is largely unknown, but the most common aetiology is X chromosome abnormalities.

Arora P, Polson DW. Diagnosis and management of premature ovarian failure. *TOG* 2011;13:67–72.

BMJ Best Practice Premature Ovarian Failure 2020,; reviewed 2023.

9. A. Ectopic pregnancy

Ectopic pregnancy is more common following transplantation due to adhesions from previous surgery and peritoneal dialysis. The miscarriage rate is similar to the general population. Whilst premature rupture of membranes and foetal growth restriction are more common in transplant recipients, oligohydramnios is not.

Kapoor N, Makanjuola D, Shehata H. Management of women with chronic renal disease in pregnancy. *TOG* 2009;11:185–91.

10. C. Spillage of a dermoid cyst

Chemical peritonitis is a rare complication arising from dermoid cyst spillage. The incidence is 0.2–8%. Long-term sequelae include pelvic adhesive disease, bowel obstruction, subfertility, abdominal wall abscesses, and fistulas.

Stavroulis A, Memtsa M, Yoong W. Methods for specimen removal from the peritoneal cavity after laparoscopic excision. *TOG* 2013;15:26–30.

11. C. 3c tear

Over 85% of women in the UK sustain a perineal injury at the time of delivery, with up to 6% experiencing third- and fourth-degree tears. Third-degree tears include disruption of the anal sphincter muscles, which are further subdivided into 3a: <50% thickness of external sphincter torn; 3b: >50% thickness of external sphincter torn; 3c: Both internal and external sphincter torn. Fourth-degree tears include disruption of the anal epithelium.

Lone F, Sultan A, Thakar R. Obstetric pelvic floor and anal sphincter injuries. *TOG* 2012;14:257–66.

RCOG Green-top Guideline 29. The management of third and fourth degree perineal tears; 2015.

12. B. 4 mm

With a 4-mm endometrial thickness cut-off, the overall sensitivity for excluding endometrial cancer was 95% and transvaginal ultrasound has >99% negative predictive value.

Bakour S, Timmermans A, Willem B, Khan K. Management of women with post-menopausal bleeding: evidence-based review. *TOG* 2012;14:243–9.

BGCS Uterine Cancer Guidelines: Recommendations for Practice 2021

13. E. Transabdominal cerclage can be performed preconceptually or in early pregnancy

Cerclage is not recommended for ultrasound-identified funnelling of the cervix in the absence of cervical shortening to 25 mm or less. Insertion of a cerclage is not recommended in women without a history of spontaneous preterm delivery or second-trimester loss who have an incidentally identified short cervix of 25 mm or less. Cerclage is not recommended in women on the basis of a history of previous cervical cone biopsy alone. Transabdominal cerclage can be performed preconceptually or in early pregnancy. Contraindications to cerclage insertion do include PPROM.

RCOG Green-top Guideline 60. Cervical cerclage; May 2011, updated as Guideline 75, 2022.

14. D. Treatment is initially imiquimod

The incidence of VIN 3 is 2 in 100,000 and it may become cancerous if left untreated. Other risk factors include multiple sexual partners, immunosuppression, smoking, and HPV 16. Treatment can include imiquimod, 5 fluorouracil cream, laser ablation, or wide local excision. Some 3–5% of women with the inflammatory disorder lichen sclerosis develop vulval cancer; 9–18.5% of women diagnosed with VIN will go on to develop squamous cell carcinoma.

BASHH 2014 UK National guideline on the management of vulval conditions.

RCOG Green-top Guideline 58. The management of vulval skin disorders; 2011.

15. B. It does not increase the risk of miscarriage

CMV is a herpes virus which is the most common cause of foetal infection. Overall, congenital CMV infection occurs in 0.2–2.2% of live births. Ultrasound features include intracranial calcification, ventriculomegaly, bowel echogenicity, and non-immune hydrops. It does not increase the risk of miscarriage, but increases the risk of IUD and stillbirth. Pyrimethamine is used to treat toxoplasmosis.

Nyberg DA, McGahan JP, Pretorius DH, Pilu G. *Diagnostic imaging of fetal anomalies.* Philadelphia: Lippincott Williams & Wilkins; 2002; pp. 746–52.

16. E. Ultrasound monitoring of the ovarian response is an integral part of the IVF treatment cycle

In women less than 40 years of age who have not conceived after two years of regular unprotected intercourse or 12 cycles of artificial insemination, offer three full cycles of IVF with or without ICSI. If the woman reaches 40 years of age during treatment, complete the current full cycle but do not offer a further full cycle. In women aged 40–42 years who have not conceived after two years of regular unprotected intercourse or 12 cycles of artificial insemination, offer one full cycle of IVF with or without ICSI, provided they have never had IVF treatment before, have no evidence of low ovarian reserve, and have discussed the additional implications of IVF and pregnancy at this age. In women aged less than 37 years or 37–39 years, consider single embryo transfer with top-quality embryos. Consider double embryo transfer if no top-quality embryos are present. In women 40–42 years, consider double embryo transfer. Ultrasound monitoring during ovarian stimulation in IVF cycles is strongly recommended to monitor the response. Do not offer natural cycle IVF treatment; use ovarian stimulation as part of IVF treatment with either urinary or recombinant gonadotrophins for ovarian stimulation part of IVF treatment.

NICE Guideline 156. Fertility: assessment and treatment for people with fertility problems; 2013, updated 2017.

17. A. A 19-year-old postnatal patient on the serenity suite (24 weeks intrauterine foetal death following prolonged prelabour rupture of membranes), feeling unwell with pyrexia and tachycardia; you note she has two red scores on MEOWS chart with reduced urinary output

Each case should be reviewed and then the order of action be prioritized. Patient D's CTG should be reviewed to decide whether vaginal delivery is imminent or whether an instrumental delivery is indicated. In that case, while patient A is being reviewed, this can be organized. Patient E will be a low priority until patient A and patient D have been dealt with. Patient C needs to be assessed later if CTG is satisfactory. In the meantime, syntocinon infusion can be continued. Patient A is a top priority as she is a case of sepsis. Her management prioritization depends on maternal well-being, starting with airway, breathing, and circulation. The recent CEMACE reports highlight the risks of sepsis as a cause of maternal mortality.

Helmreich RL. On error management: lessons from aviation. *BMJ* 2000;320:781–5.

Lewis G, ed. *Saving mothers' lives: the seventh report of the confidential enquiries into maternal deaths in the United Kingdom.* London: CEMECH; 2007.

18. B. Crown rump length of 7 mm with an absent foetal heartbeat

Ultrasound diagnosis of miscarriage should only be considered with a mean gestation sac diameter of 25 mm or more (with no obvious yolk sac), or with a foetal pole with crown rump length of 7 mm or more with no foetal heart activity. Here it is important to seek a second opinion on the viability of the pregnancy and/or perform a second scan a minimum of 7 days after the first before making a diagnosis.

NICE Guideline 126. Ectopic pregnancy and miscarriage: diagnosis and initial management; 2019, updated 2021.

19. B. Calcium channel blockers

Nifedipine has been shown to delay birth for up to seven days and is associated with improved neonatal outcomes when compared to beta-agonists, although there are no data on long-term outcomes. It is unlicensed for use as a tocolytic. Magnesium sulphate is commonly used in the US for tocolysis but is rarely used for this indication in the UK. Beta-agonists have known tocolytic properties. Ritodrine is no longer recommended for this use in the UK. These drugs have a high frequency of maternal adverse effects, including palpitations, tremor, nausea, or vomiting, headache, chest pain, and dyspnoea. Atosiban, an oxytocin receptor agonist, is comparable to nifedipine in delaying birth for up to seven days and may be considered as an alternative to nifedipine.

NICE Guideline 25. Preterm labour and birth; 2015.

20. A. Dietary factors, such as poor intake of vitamin A, are linked to complete molar pregnancies

Complete molar pregnancies are generally diploid, with the genetic material being paternally derived. Partial moles are usually (90%) triploid in karyotype resulting from dispermic fertilization of a normal ovum. A deficiency of vitamin A, or carotene, is associated with a higher incidence of complete mole. Extremes of age, Asian and Japanese ethnicity, and previous gestational trophoblastic disease are risk factors for molar pregnancy. Less than 1 in 200 molar pregnancies are twin pregnancies and can lead to a successful outcome in approximately one-third of cases. After appropriate counselling, the pregnancy can be allowed to continue. There is a 0.5% chance of requiring chemotherapy after a partial mole. Following chemotherapy, conception should be avoided for one year. If no chemotherapy is required, and HCG levels are normal within 56 days, follow-up is completed by six months from the date of surgical evacuation and the couple can attempt a further pregnancy.

Berkowitz RS, et al. Risk factors for a complete molar pregnancy forms case control study. *Am J Obstet Gynecol* 1985;152(8):1016–20.

RCOG Green-top Guideline 38. The management of gestational trophoblastic disease; 2010, 4th ed., 2020.

Savage P. Molar pregnancy. *TOG* 2008;10:3–8.

21. C. Family history of thromboembolism

All the risk factors previously identified are well recognized, including obesity, complicated heart disease, and GTN. Contraceptives are metabolized in the liver and a liver tumour is an obvious contraindication. UK Medical Eligibility Criteria (UKMEC) categories are used to provide guidance for clinicians prescribing contraceptive methods. There are four categories ranging from unrestricted use (category 1) to unacceptable health risks and should not be used (category 4).

Gestational trophoblastic neoplasia with an abnormal HCG is UKMEC category 4. BMI 35–39 kg/m^2 is UKMEC category 3; BMI ≥40 kg/m^2 is category 4. Valvular and congenital heart disease complicated by pulmonary hypertension, atrial fibrillation, or history of subacute bacterial endocarditis is UKMEC category 4. Family history in first-degree relative aged <45 years is UKMEC category 3. Benign or malignant liver tumours is UKMEC category 4.

Faculty of Family Planning & Reproductive Healthcare Clinical Effectiveness Unit Guidance. The UK Medical Eligibility Criteria for contraceptive use; 2009, 2016 amended 2019.

22. A. A banana-shaped cerebellum is seen on ultrasound scan in more than 99% of cases

Myelomeningecele is a severe congenital malformation of the central nervous system which results from incomplete closure of the neural tube during the third to fourth week of embryonic development. It is characterized by a malformation of the spinal cord and a defect in the posterior spinal elements and overlying skin. Hydrocephalous is present in more than 70% of cases. Ventriculomegaly and the so-called lemon sign, defined as scalloping of the frontal bones of the foetal skull are also common.

Kumar S. *Handbook of fetal medicine*. Cambridge: Cambridge University Press; 2010; p. 41.

Kunpalin Y, et al. Cranial findings detected by second-trimester ultrasound in fetuses with myelomeningecele: a systematic review. *BJOG* 2021;128(2):366–74.

23. A. All HIV-positive women should attend for annual cytology with an initial colposcopy

All women in England and Ireland are invited for three yearly smear tests between ages 25 and 55 years. They are invited for five yearly smears (if all previous results have been normal) from 55 to 65 years. In Scotland and Wales, women are invited for three yearly smears from age 20 to 60. The reason for this lack of consensus is a lack of robust evidence to dictate best practice. CIN develops from the basement membrane of the epithelial layer and therefore CIN 1 affects the basal (lower) third of the epithelial layer, CIN 2 affects the lower two-thirds, and CIN 3 affects the full thickness of the epithelial layer. Cancer is diagnosed when the abnormal cells invade through the basement membrane.

CIN 1 resolves spontaneously in the majority (80%) of patients as the HPV virus is cleared. Only a small percentage of CIN 1 persists and even fewer cases progress to high-grade CIN. Progression to invasive disease takes on average 15 years and is usually in a stepwise fashion (from CIN 1, to CIN 2, to CIN 3 before invasion occurs). Treating all cases of CIN 1 would result in massive overtreatment and unnecessary exposure of low-risk women to treatment.

Even treatment with local destructive (cold coagulation, laser ablation, cryotherapy) has been associated with short- and long-term consequences. The risks of long-term complications of stenosis and incompetence are not thought to be as high as those associated with LLETZ (excisional treatment) but are still increased in comparison to no treatment. Further research is ongoing to quantify these risks.

HIV-positive women are immunosuppressed (as a side effect of the anti-retroviral therapy) and therefore the risk of persistent HPV is greater. This can result in a higher incidence of CIN with resulting progression to high-grade CIN or invasion and therefore this group of women are encouraged to attend for an annual smear with an initial colposcopy if resources permit.

NHSCSP Document 20. English colposcopy guidelines: recommendations and standards; 3rd ed.; 2016.

24. B. In the last MBRRACE-UK Confidential Enquiry, the commonest cause of direct deaths in the UK was due to thrombosis and thromboembolism

Maternal mortality rate in the UK is defined as the number of direct and indirect deaths per 100,000 maternities. The direct maternal death rate rose significantly between 2015–17 and 2018–20. Maternities are defined as the number of pregnancies that result in a live birth at any gestation or stillbirths occurring at or after 24 completed weeks of gestation, and are required to be notified by law. In the last MBRRACE-UK Confidential Enquiry, the commonest cause of direct deaths in the UK was due to thrombosis and thromboembolism. There remains a more than three-fold difference in maternal mortality rates among women from Black ethnic backgrounds. Globally, the maternal mortality ratio has decreased by 34%. The Millennium Development Goal 5 is a pledge by the World Health Organization to help developing countries to improve their health system in order to improve women's health.

MBRRACE-UK Saving Lives, Improving Mothers Care; 2022.

World Health Organization. *Beyond the numbers: reviewing maternal deaths and complications to make pregnancy safer.* Geneva: WHO; 2004.

World Health Organization. *Trends in maternal mortality: 1990 to 2008.* Geneva: WHO; 2010.

25. A. An ovarian cyst over 10 cm in maximal diameter

The IOTA group ultrasound 'rules' to classify masses as benign include the following features: unilocular cysts, solid components (largest diameter <7 mm), acoustic shadowing, smooth multilocular tumour, largest diameter <100 mm, and no blood flow. The features which may indicate malignancy include irregular solid tumours, the presence of ascites, a minimum of four papillary structures, irregular multilocular solid tumours with largest diameter of over 100 mm, with very strong blood flow.

RCOG Green-top Guideline 62. Management of suspected ovarian masses; 2011.

26. C. Colles' fascia

Extension of bleeding in the anterior triangle is limited by Colles' fascia and the urogenital diaphragm, while the anal fascia limits the extension of bleeding in the posterior triangle.

StratOG. Management of labour and delivery, perioperative trauma, para-genital haematomas.

27. A. All women should have commenced combined antiretroviral therapy by week 24 of pregnancy

Although pregnancy has no clear effect on HIV progression, all pregnant HIV-positive women should be advised to take combined antiretroviral therapy (cART) during pregnancy, including elite controllers. Without treatment, HIV is vertically transmitted in approximately 25% of cases. A regime of tenofovir or abacavir with emtricitabine or lamivudine as a nucleoside backbone is recommended in the first instance. Zidovudine monotherapy is not recommended and should only be used in women declining cART with a viral load of <10,000 HIV RNA copies/mL and willing to have a caesarean section.

BHIVA Guideline for the management of HIV infection in pregnancy and postpartum; 2012 (2014 interim review); 2018 (2020 third interim update).

RCOG Green-top Guideline 39. HIV in pregnancy; 2010. (NB: this is now archived)

28. E. Women undergoing an operative vaginal delivery are less likely to report difficulty in conceiving and more likely to have a further pregnancy than those who undergo a CS

CS at full dilatation is associated with more than double the risk of intraoperative trauma. The risk of wound infection is low regardless of the route of delivery. The frequency of constipation is higher at one year with assisted vaginal delivery.

Vousden N, et al. Caesarean section at full dilatation: incidence, impact and current management. *TOG* 2014;16:199–205.

29. E. Primigravida and maternal age 42

NICE recommends that low-dose aspirin is reserved for high-risk patients or patients with two moderate risk factors. Moderate risk factors include primigravida, age above 40 years, pregnancy interval greater than ten years, family history of pre-eclampsia, multiple pregnancy, and BMI over 35 kg/m^2 at booking. Here women should take 75–150 mg of aspirin from 12 weeks until the birth of the baby. Major risk factors include hypertensive disease in a previous pregnancy, chronic kidney disease, autoimmune disease, diabetes, and chronic hypertension. In these cases, 75 mg of aspirin should be prescribed from 12 weeks gestation until delivery.

Mone F, McAuliffe FM. Low-dose aspirin and calcium supplementation for the prevention of pre-eclampsia. *TOG* 2014;16:245–50.

NICE Guideline CG133. Hypertension in pregnancy: diagnosis and management; 2019.

30. E. Regional anaesthesia is not contraindicated for delivery for placenta praevia or suspected placenta accreta

Grey-scale ultrasound complemented by colour Doppler and three-dimensional power Doppler remains the imaging modality of choice with sensitivity of up to 100% and specificity of up to 85%. This should be performed at 32 weeks gestation and in asymptomatic women, an additional ultrasound is recommended at 36 weeks gestation to inform discussion around the mode of delivery. MRI may also be used to assess the depth of invasion and lateral extension of myometrial invasion, especially with posterior placentation and/or suspected parametrial invasion. The value of prophylactic placement of arterial catheters at the time of delivery for suspected cases of placenta accreta remains unclear and should be assessed on an individual basis. Regional anaesthesia is not contraindicated for delivery for placenta praevia or suspected placenta accreta. This is usually decided in a multidisciplinary approach. The use of methotrexate in such situations remains unclear and it is not recommended for routine administration.

RCOG Green-top Guideline. 27a. Placenta praevia and placenta accreta: diagnosis and management; 2018.

RCOG Green-top Guideline. 52. Prevention and management of postpartum haemorrhage; 2009.

31. E. Phaeochromocytoma

Open spina bifida, cleft lip, exomphalous, serious cardiac anomalies, lethal skeletal dysplasia, and trisomy 13 and 18 are also included in the list of conditions which are screened for.

NHS Fetal Anomaly Screening Programme 2013–2014; updated 2021.

32. A. Cystic fibrosis is transmitted as an autosomal recessive disease

Increasing numbers of women with cystic fibrosis are reaching childbearing age. If the partner is shown to be a carrier for the cystic fibrosis gene, chorionic villus sampling or amniocentesis may be offered for this autosomal recessive disease. Factor VII deficiency is an autosomal recessive disease. It is rare, affecting 1 in 500,000 births. Marfan's syndrome, neurofibromatosis type 1, and Huntington's disease are all autosomal dominant diseases.

Firth HV, Hurst JA. *Clinical genetics.* Oxford: Oxford Desk Reference; 2006.

McGowan B. *Obstetrics and gynaecology,* 3rd ed. London: Churchill Livingstone; 2005. Ch. 1: Prenatal diagnosis.

33. A. Copper intrauterine device

The copper IUD is the only emergency contraception (EC) that is not affected by liver enzyme-inducing drugs or HIV post-exposure. If the copper IUD is not available or acceptable, the woman should be advised to take two levonorgestrel tablets (3 mg), however the effectiveness of this regimen is unknown. It is important to ask about the use of liver enzyme-inducing drugs currently and within the last 28 days as both affect the efficacy of EC.

Faculty of Sexual and Reproductive Healthcare Clinical Guidance. Emergency contraception: drug interactions with hormonal contraception; updated 2012, 2020.

34. E. Routine follow-up is not required and the patient should be reassured

CA125 is not required unless there are complex features or the woman is postmenopausal. The patient can be discharged and reassured if the ovarian cyst is found to be simple and less than 5 cm in size, with no symptoms. If torsion is suspected and a cyst is confirmed, prompt laparoscopic assessment and untwisting of the pedicle may rescue the ovary.

RCOG/BSGE Joint Green-top Guideline 62. Management of suspected ovarian masses in premenopausal women; November 2011.

35. D. Obesity

Risk factors for endometrial cancer include early menarche, late menopause, nulliparity, use of HRT over five years, obesity, tamoxifen therapy, family history, granulosa cell tumours, PCOS, and age. Cigarette smoking is significantly associated with a reduced risk of endometrial cancer.

Zhou B, et al. Cigarette smoking and the risk of endometrial cancer: a meta-analysis. *Am J Med* 2008;121(6):501–8.

36. D. Specialist physiotherapy

It can improve symptoms in 60% of cases and the evidence shows that pelvic floor muscle training is just as effective as surgery for around half of women with stress urinary incontinence. Supervised pelvic floor muscle training should be offered for at least 3 months' duration in the first instance for women with stress or mixed urinary incontinence.

NICE Clinical Guideline 123. Urinary incontinence and pelvic organ prolapse in women: management; 2019.

37. A. 50 μg per vagina four hourly

The RCOG Green-top Guidelines recommend adjusting the misoprostol dose to the gestational age. Before a gestational age of 26 weeks, 100 μg six hourly should be prescribed, and 25–50 μg four hourly for a gestational age of 27 weeks or more. Misoprostol can also be used in women with one previous caesarean section, but lower doses should be considered.

Nzewi C, Araklitis G, Narvekar N. The use of mifepristone and misoprostol in the management of late intrauterine fetal death. *TOG* 2014;16:233–8.

RCOG Green-top Guideline 55. Late intrauterine fetal death and stillbirth; 2010.

38. B. Hysteroscopic resection of submucous fibroid

Tranexamic acid will not correct the cause of her bleeding. As she would like to conceive, the Mirena intrauterine system, uterine artery embolization, or endometrial resection will not be acceptable.

NICE Clinical Guideline 88. Heavy menstrual bleeding: assessment and management; 2007, 2018, updated 2021.

39. C. If the result of the first semen analysis is suboptimal, a repeat test is recommended after three months with encouragement for healthy lifestyle changes

The term 'mild male factor infertility' is extensively used in the literature and in clinical practice. It is defined as two or more semen analyses with one or more variables below the 5th centile (as defined by WHO). According to WHO 2013, a semen analysis is considered normal if a count of 15 million per ml, motility of 40%, and morphology of 4% or more of normal forms are present. The sperm production cycle takes 12 weeks, so if the semen analysis result is suboptimal then encourage the male to make healthy lifestyle changes and to repeat the test after three months. In cases of severe oligospermia or azoospermia, repeat the test as soon as possible. Screening for anti-sperm antibodies should not be offered as there is no evidence for any effective treatment to improve fertility. There is no evidence that post-coital cervical mucous testing has any predictive value in improving pregnancy, so it is not recommended in routine fertility investigations.

NICE Clinical Guideline 156. Assessment and treatment for people with fertility problems; 2013; updated 2017.

40. C. Infection rate is similar regardless of whether medical, surgical, or expectant management is undertaken

Conservative management has an average success rate of 50%. Mifepristone should not be offered as a treatment for missed or incomplete miscarriage. Anti-D is not routinely required for women who miscarry naturally under 12 weeks gestation, but is indicated in ectopic or molar pregnancy, therapeutic termination of pregnancy and in cases of uterine bleeding where this is repeated, heavy or associated with abdominal pain.

NICE Clinical Guideline 126. Ectopic pregnancy and miscarriage: diagnosis and initial management; 2012, 2019; updated 2021.

41. D. Over 50% of significant (>4 ml) fetomaternal haemorrhages will occur during normal vaginal delivery

Anti-D immunoglobulin is recommended in all Rhesus-negative women with spontaneous miscarriage after 12 weeks. It is also recommended at any gestation in those who have surgical evacuation of the uterus. It should be considered in women undergoing medical intervention. Anti-D immunoglobulin should be given to all Rhesus-negative women with ectopic pregnancy regardless of management. Anti-D immunoglobulin should ideally be administered into the deltoid muscle. Administration into the gluteus muscle may penetrate only subcutaneously and therefore lead to delayed absorption. Anti-D immunoglobulin should be given within 72 hours of the event in women with persistent vaginal bleeding after 20 weeks gestation. If the bleed is large, or no cause found, Kleihauer testing can be carried out at two-week intervals to test for the size of the haemorrhage. Whilst a traumatic delivery is a risk factor for fetomaternal haemorrhage, over 50% occur during normal delivery. Risk factors for fetomaternal haemorrhage include miscarriage, threatened miscarriage, delivery, manual removal of the placenta, stillbirth and foetal death, abdominal trauma, multiple pregnancies (at delivery), and in-utero therapeutic interventions. Approximately 3% of deliveries will have a fetomaternal haemorrhage >15 ml and so will need additional anti-D immunoglobulin. It is recommended to quantify the size of the fetomaternal haemorrhage in Rhesus-D mothers within two hours of delivery in order to identify the women who will need additional prophylaxis.

Qureshi H, et al. BSCH guideline for the use of anti-D immunoglobulin for the prevention of haemolytic disease of the fetus and newborn. *Transfus Med* 2014:24:8–20.

RCOG Green-top Guideline 22. The use of anti-D immunoglobulin for Rhesus D prophylaxis; 2011 (archived).

42. A. The time limit for detection of body fluids in the vagina following digital penetration is 12 hours

The time limit for the detection of body fluids, cellular material, or lubricants on the skin is 48 hours. The time limit for detection of semen in the mouth is 48 hours following oral penetration. The time limit for detection of semen in the rectum following anal penetration is 72 hours (three days). Foreign trace material can be identified on skin swabs for 48 hours, and in certain circumstances, up to one week. Semen can be detected in the vagina for up to seven days.

Wyatt JP. *Oxford handbook of forensic medicine.* Oxford: Oxford University Press; 2011.

43. D. 8%

Women should be informed that spontaneous version is unusual at term and occurs in only 8% of primigravid women after 36 weeks gestation. For women who have a failed attempt at ECV, 3–7% of babies spontaneously turn to cephalic presentation. Spontaneous reversion to breech after a successful ECV is rare, occurring in 3%. However, it is recommended that an ultrasound scan be performed prior to performing a planned elective CS for breech presentation.

NICE and National Guideline Alliance NG201. Antenatal care: management of breech presentation; 2021.

RCOG Green-top Guideline 20a. External cephalic version and reducing the incidence of term breech presentation; 2006; updated 2017.

44. B. Foetal alloimmune thrombocytopenia is a relative contraindication to operative vaginal delivery

Suspected foetal bleeding disorders or a predisposition to fracture are relative contraindications to assisted vaginal delivery. In primiparous women with an epidural, there is insufficient evidence to recommend starting oxytocin in the second stage of labour as a strategy to reduce the need for assisted delivery. One of the criteria for midcavity forceps is that the foetal head is no more than one-fifth palpable per abdomen. Vacuum delivery should be avoided below 32 weeks gestation and considered with caution between 32 weeks + 0 days and 36 weeks + 0 days gestation. Maternal BMI greater than 30 has been shown to increase the rate of failed instrumental delivery.

RCOG Green-top Guideline 26. Assisted vaginal birth 2020; originally operative vaginal delivery; 2011.

45. B. Multidisciplinary assistance is needed when initial crystalloid and colloid therapy fails, leading to persistent haemoconcentration and dehydration

Paracentesis should be considered in women who are distressed due to abdominal distension, experience shortness of breath and respiratory compromise, or in whom oliguria persists despite adequate volume replacement. It will help to keep fluid in intravascular compartments. After paracentesis, replace fluid with colloids to elevate the intra-abdominal pressure and increase renal perfusion. Multidisciplinary assistance is needed when initial crystalloid and colloid therapy fails, leading to persistent haemoconcentration and dehydration. If the condition starts deteriorating it involves other organs as well, so anaesthetic and medical colleagues may be required to help in the management of resistant severe OHSS and critical OHSS; patients may need intensive-care monitoring in rare cases. Diuretics should not be used in women with oliguria secondary to a reduced blood volume and decreased renal perfusion, as they may worsen intravascular dehydration. However, they may have a role with careful haemodynamic monitoring in cases where oliguria persists despite adequate intravascular volume expansion and a normal intra-abdominal pressure. Pelvic surgery should be restricted to cases with adnexal torsion or co-incident problems requiring surgery, and undertaken only by an experienced surgeon following careful assessment. It is not recommended to reduce the size of ovaries. Women should be reassured that pregnancy may continue normally despite OHSS, and there is no evidence of an increased risk of congenital abnormalities. In very rare scenarios, termination of pregnancy is needed. In IVF cycles if OHSS is noted, then embryo transfer is usually deferred to the next cycle, giving time to resolve OHSS.

RCOG Green-top Guideline 5. The management of ovarian hyperstimulation syndrome; 2006; updated 2016.

46. D. Previous caesarean section for foetal malpresentation

Epidural anaesthesia is not contraindicated in a planned VBAC, although the evidence of the likelihood of a successful VBAC is variable and frequent epidural dosing may be an independent risk factor for impending uterine rupture in VBAC labour. VBAC at or after 41 weeks of gestation decreases the likelihood of a successful VBAC. Successful VBAC is more likely in women with previous caesarean section for foetal malpresentation (84%) compared with women who have had a caesarean section for either labour dystocia (64%) or foetal distress (73%). Previous caesarean section for induced labour, no previous vaginal birth, and BMI >30 all decrease the likelihood of a successful VBAC. When all these factors are present together, the success rate is 40% compared to the overall success rate of 72–76%.

RCOG Green-top Guideline 45. Birth after previous caesarean section; 2007, updated 2015.

47. C. Expectant management

85% of women with an intrauterine foetal death will labour spontaneously within three weeks of diagnosis. If there is no evidence of ruptured membranes, pre-eclampsia, infection, or bleeding, the risk of expectant management for 48 hours is low. There is, however, a 10% chance of maternal DIC within four weeks of the date of foetal death. The addition of mifepristone to a misoprostol regime has been proven to reduce the average duration of labour when compared with regimes not including mifepristone. Intrapartum administration of intravenous antibiotics for carriers of group B Streptococcus is primarily intended to reduce the risk of neonatal infection, not maternal.

NICE Clinical Guideline 70. Induction of labour; 2008.

48. D. Risk factors include immunosuppression

The incidence of VIN 3 is 2 in 100,000. Other risk factors include multiple sexual partners, immunosuppression, smoking, and HPV 16. Treatment can include imiquimod, vulvectomy, laser ablation, or wide local excision. Some 3–5% of women with the inflammatory disorder lichen sclerosis develop vulval cancer; 4% of women diagnosed with VIN will have intraepithelial neoplasia at other lower genital tract sites.

BASSH Guidelines. Skin conditions of the vulva; 2014.

Cullis P, Mudzamiri T, Millan D, Siddiqui N. Vulval intraepithelial neoplasia: making sense of the literature. *TOG* 2011;13:73–8.

Kingston A. The postmenopausal vulva. *TOG* 2009;11:253–9.

RCOG Guidelines for the diagnosis and management of vulval carcinoma; 2014.

49. C. Hysterectomy is a definitive cure for heavy menstrual bleeding associated with fibroids

Tranexamic acid has no effect on the size of fibroid. High-dose oral progestogen has no effect on the size of the fibroid. Hysterectomy is a definitive treatment for fibroids and heavy menstrual bleeding. Endometrial ablation has no effect on the size of the fibroid. A levonorgestrel-containing IUS may decrease the size of fibroid by 30% and may be considered as the first-line treatment for heavy menstrual bleeding in women with fibroids less than 3 cm in diameter which do not distort the uterine cavity.

NICE Clinical Guideline 88. Heavy menstrual bleeding: assessment and management; 2018, updated 2021.

50. A. Frequency and nocturia

Frequency and nocturia indicate a bladder storage problem. The International Continence Society classifies symptoms into three groups: those that indicate abnormal *storage* (stress incontinence, urge incontinence, frequency, nocturia, nocturnal enuresis), abnormal *voiding* (hesitance, incomplete emptying, poor stream, post-micturition dribble, straining to void), and abnormal *sensation* (urgency, dysuria, painful bladder, loin pain, absent sensation).

RCOG, commissioned by NICE. Urinary incontinence in women: the management of urinary incontinence in women; 2013; updated 2019.

Extended Matching Questions

Answers for Questions 1–5

1. J; 2. G; 3. D; 4. C; 5. K

1. Pneumothorax can develop post-delivery after an active second stage. The signs of reduced air entry and a hyper-resonant percussion note should aid in diagnosis. Chest X-ray is mandatory to confirm this.

2. Peripartum cardiomyopathy is rare and typically the patient is multiparous and the presentation is during the postnatal period. Antenatal presentations can also occur. Pulmonary embolism would need to be ruled out with such presentations, but the presence of biventricular failure with pulmonary oedema helps in the diagnosis.

3. Hyperventilation is not an uncommon presentation in pregnancy. It typically presents with shortness of breath associated with paraesthesia of hands and mouth. The key to diagnosis is the presence of normal saturations in room air, but an arterial blood gas showing hypocapnia.

4. The diagnosis is diabetic ketoacidosis, which is associated with a clinical presentation of feeling unwell, lethargy, and laboured deep respiration (Kussmaul breathing) in an insulin-dependent diabetic. It may be associated with infection, poor glycaemic control, and insulin therapy, resulting in high blood glucose.

5. Women admitted with OHSS are at higher risk of developing DVT and Pes due to dehydration. There is no sign of clinical infection here.

Nelson-Piercy C. *Obstetric medicine*, 6th ed. Boca Raton: CRC Press; 2020.

Answers for Questions 6–10

6. I; 7. H; 8. I; 9. H; 10. B

6. Woman who are known to have an asymptomatic thrombophilia excluding antithrombin deficiency, combined defects, and homozygous for factor V Leiden, with one other risk factors should be considered for at least 10 days of prophylactic dose LMWH postnatally. Here, whilst the patient is heterozygous for factor V Leiden, her age is also a risk factor.

7. Women who are known to have a high-risk asymptomatic thrombophilia such as combined defects and homozygous for factor V Leiden, but no history of thromboembolism should be considered for antenatal and six weeks postnatal prophylactic dose LMWH.

8. All women with a BMI above 40 kg/m^2 prepregnancy or in early pregnancy should be considered for ten days' LMWH at a weight-adjusted prophylactic dose postnatally.

9. Women who have had an oestrogen-provoked venous thromboembolism (the contraceptive pill or pregnancy) should be considered for antenatal and postnatal prophylactic dose LMWH, for at least six weeks after delivery.

10. Women known to have antiphopholipid syndrome and have a previous history of venous thromboembolism are at very high risk and therefore require a high-dose LMWH antenatally and postnatally in addition to long-term anticoagulation. Management should be in collaboration with a haematologist with expertise in thrombosis in pregnancy.

RCOG Green-top Guideline 37a. Reducing the risk of venous thromboembolism during pregnancy and the puerperium; 2009; updated 2015.

Answers for Questions 11–15

11. C; 12. N; 13. C; 14. F; 15. C

11. People with SLE are at an increased risk of ischaemic heart disease, stroke, and venous thromboembolism. The Faculty of Sexual and Reproductive Health (FSRH) advises that all combined hormonal methods should be avoided. CHC = UKMEC 4; progestogen-only methods and IUS = UKMEC 2.

12. The use of hormonal contraceptives including combined hormonal methods is not considered to exacerbate viral hepatitis or mild compensated liver cirrhosis without complications. For carriers of viral hepatitis, it appears that hormonal contraceptive use does not trigger liver failure or severe dysfunction. UKMEC = 1.

13. The UKMEC classifies having a first-degree relative with a history of VTE under the age of 45 years as a UKMEC 3 for CHC because of the small possibility of a hereditary predisposition. A negative thrombophilia screen does not necessarily exclude all thrombogenic mutations.

14. Some contraceptives (traditional POP, copper IUD, levonorgestrel-containing IUS) are associated with an increased risk of ectopic pregnancy risk if the method fails. However, all contraceptive methods prevent pregnancies and thus protect against ectopic pregnancies as well. In this case, all intrauterine contraception = UKMEC 13, due to the distortion of the uterine cavity by the fibroids.

15. CHC = UKMEC 3. The major concerns are vascular disease due to diabetes and additional risk of arterial thrombosis due to combined hormonal contraceptive use. It should be noted that with neuropathy/retinopathy, progestogen-only injectables (Depo-Provera®) are WHO MEC 3, but UKMEC 2. For the purposes of the MRCOG Part 2 exam, we would recommend relying on the UKMEC, although there is concern regarding hypo-oestrogenic effects and reduced HDL levels among users of Depo-Provera. The effects may persist for some time after discontinuation. Some POCs may increase the risk of arterial thrombosis, although this increase is substantially less than with CHC. Other progestogen-only methods such as the POP or progestogen implant have not been shown to have an adverse effect on HDL levels.

Faculty of Sexual & Reproductive Health (FSRH). UK Medical Eligibility Criteria for contraceptive use UKMEC; 2016; amended 2019.

WHO. *Medical eligibility criteria for contraceptive use*, 5th ed.; 2015.

Answers for Questions 16–20

16. J; 17. M; 18. G; 19. A; 20. L

16. In stage 4A the carcinoma has spread beyond the true pelvis involving adjacent organs or there has been biopsy proven spread to the bladder or rectal mucosa.

17. CIN 3 is not cervical cancer and therefore is not staged using the FIGO staging system.

18. In stage 2B the carcinoma has spread beyond the uterus and involves the parametrium but not the pelvic side or lower third of the vagina.

19. In stage 1A1 the carcinoma is confined to the cervix or corpus uteri. It is microscopic, with a measured maximal stromal invasion of 3.0 mm in depth and an extension of 7.0 mm.

20. No information has been given on examination and investigations to exclude possible spread, such as an examination under anaesthesia, cystoscopy, proctoscopy, intravenous urography, and X-rays.

FIGO. Revised FIGO staging for carcinoma of the vulva, cervix, and endometrium. *Int J Gynecol Obstet* 2009;105:103–4.

Answers for Questions 21–25

21. K; 22. B; 23. A; 24. H; 25. F

21. This patient is acutely unwell and appears to be deteriorating. The most appropriate plan of management is for urgent transfer to ITU for stabilization.
22. Any new onset chest pain and shortness of breath should be investigated to exclude cardiac or respiratory causes such as thrombosis; hence an arterial blood gas is the most appropriate immediate next step.
23. Given this woman is showing clinical signs of sepsis, antibiotics are the most appropriate management.
24. As both mother and foetus are tachycardic with maternal pyrexia, urgent delivery is needed to minimize the exposure of the baby to sepsis.
25. Crystalloid infusion is needed to manage this woman's fluid balance, given she is in septic and haemorrhagic shock.

RCOG Green-top Guidelines 64a, 64b. Bacterial sepsis in pregnancy; bacterial sepsis following pregnancy; 2012.

Answers for Questions 26–30

26. L; 27. G; 28. B; 29. J; 30. E

26. Pelvic sepsis should be considered with a delayed presentation on day five following delivery. Patients with prolonged labour, high BMI, and prolonged rupture of membranes are at risk. The key factor here is the presence of pyrexia and pelvic pain but no vomiting.
27. Group A Streptococcus infection is a cause of maternal mortality, and a respiratory rate of over 20 per minute is a key point. It can cause a range of infections, from superficial skin infections to cellulitis, pneumonia, and toxic shock syndrome.
28. The main differential here is cystitis, but a prolonged second stage followed by an instrumental delivery with signs of sepsis (rigors) is more suggestive of pyelonephritis.
29. A thorough clinical assessment is important and an inflamed breast directs you to the diagnosis.
30. Obesity, Caucasian ethnicity, female sex, and age are key risk factors for developing gallstones and cholecystitis. The key here is upper abdominal pain.

NICE Clinical Guidance 194. Postnatal care; 2021.

Answers for Questions 31–35

31. B; 32. E; 33. J; 34. G; 35. K

31. Beneficence involves balancing the benefits of treatment against the risks and costs involved.
32. Confidentiality is defined as when one person discloses information to another when it is reasonable to expect that information will be held in confidence. The GMC advises that confidentiality can be breached when it is required to do so by law and is in the public interest.
33. Non-maleficence is a principle of bioethics that asserts an obligation not to inflict harm intentionally. This principle is useful in dealing with difficult issues surrounding the terminally or seriously ill and injured.
34. The Fraser guidelines state the importance of respecting the patient's view about a particular treatment.
35. Paternalism is defined as the interference with or failure to respect affairs normally designated as matters within an individual's sphere of liberty for the sake of that individual.

RCOG. Law and ethics in relation to court-authorised obstetric intervention; 2006.

Answers for Questions 36–40

36. B; 37. D; 38. E; 39. L; 40. I

36. Case-controlled: a study which compares the outcome of cases with different methodologies. This is usually retrospective.
37. Cohort: a study which follows through a set group of patients and is usually therefore prospective.
38. Crossover design: a study in which treatments are switched over during the research period.
39. Retrospective: a study which reviews cases which have already occurred over a set period of time.
40. Prospective: a study which recruits new cases which fit the inclusion criteria and follows their outcomes. Prospective studies usually have fewer potential sources of bias and confounding than retrospective studies.

RCOG. Strat OG—Research module.

Answers for Questions 41–45

41. C; 42. J; 43. N; 44. D; 45. F

41. The RCOG's most recent clinical guideline suggests that the products of conception from a third miscarriage should be sent away for cytogenetic studies. However, it appears that in this woman's case no such action has been taken. If there is confirmed evidence of five miscarriages (with ultrasound scan or chorionic villi seen at uterine curettage) and no cytogenetic studies done so far, then there is a strong case for cytogenetic studies for this couple.
42. IVF may be considered in her case by using a modified ovarian stimulation method, although with her low AMH her response to ovarian stimulation may be suboptimal. IVF with young donor oocytes may be another option.
43. An autosomal recessive single gene disorder does not require pre-implantation embryo biopsy. Given the patient's age, in keeping with the NICE guideline, she should continue her efforts with regular unprotected sexual intercourse.
44. Once ovulation and tubal patency has been confirmed, then this couple should be offered donor insemination.
45. Well-controlled diabetic patients should be advised to take a higher dose of folic acid (5 mg daily) to reduce risk of foetal developmental abnormalities in first trimester.

NICE Clinical Guideline 156. Assessment and treatment for people with fertility problems; 2013; updated 2017.

RCOG Green-top Guideline 17. Recurrent miscarriage: investigations and treatment of couples; 2011.

Answers for Questions 46–50

46. K; 47. O; 48. L; 49. N; 50. A

46. This patient requires reassurance as the chance of miscarriage in her next pregnancy is low and all her investigations are normal.
47. A woman with a high BMI should be encouraged to lose weight in conjunction with cycle monitoring in the first instance.
48. As this patient has had more than three pregnancy losses, she should be offered thrombophilia screening as incidence of lupus anticoagulant positive antibodies is over 10% compared to its occurrence of 2% in the background population.
49. This patient possibly has a higher chance of having cervical incompetence. Vaginal and cervical swabs should be done to exclude any infections in the vagina. Once pregnant, she

should be offered a cervical length assessment. If cervical length is less than 2.5 cm even during early pregnancy, or if there is evidence of funnelling of the cervical canal, she should be offered cervical cerclage.

50. This is an open-ended question and does not say what type of abnormality was found, which can happen in clinical practice. Both partners should be offered chromosomal analysis to ensure there is no increased risk related to chromosome abnormality in either of them. This finding may have implications for future pregnancies as well.

RCOG Green-top Guideline 17. The investigation and treatment of couples with recurrent first-trimester and second-trimester miscarriage; 2011.

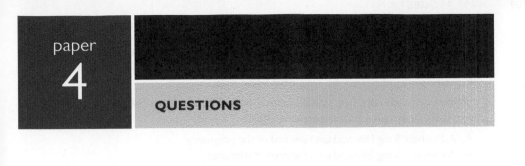
Single Best Answers

1. Upon reviewing a 28-year-old pregnant woman, you notice that she is documented to smoke 15 cigarettes a day. Which one of the following is not associated with smoking in pregnancy?

    A. Ectopic pregnancy
    B. Placenta praevia
    C. Placental abruption
    D. Pre-eclampsia
    E. Preterm delivery

2. You are organizing a VQ scan for a pregnant patient who is being investigated for shortness of breath.

    Which one of the following is the commonest teratogenic effect of exposure to high-dose radiation?

    A. Cardiac defects
    B. Central nervous system changes
    C. Foetal growth restriction
    D. Miscarriage
    E. Peripheral limb malformations

3. You are reviewing the medication of a woman who consults you for emergency contraception 24 hours after unprotected sexual intercourse. Which one of the following medications can the administered along with the levonorgestrel pill?

    A. Griseofulvin
    B. Phenytoin
    C. Rifampicin
    D. St John's wort
    E. Warfarin

4. **A 23-year-old primiparous woman is seen in an antenatal clinic at ten weeks gestation. She is known to have epilepsy, for which she takes lamotrigine. Her last fit was one year ago.**

    When considering her medication, which one of the following is the most appropriate management plan?

    A. Administer 5 mg folic acid until the end of the pregnancy
    B. Administer 5 mg folic acid until the second trimester
    C. Administer vitamin K until the end of the pregnancy
    D. Change her medication to carbamazepine
    E. Stop administering lamotrigine

5. **A 19-year-old woman presents with a one-year history of dysmenorrhoea. Which one of the following is a risk factor for dysmenorrhoea?**

    A. Early menarche
    B. Intramural fibroids
    C. Long menstrual cycle length
    D. Multiparity
    E. Ulcerative colitis

6. **A 42-year-old woman presents in her first pregnancy with monochorionic twins at ten weeks gestation. She is worried about the increased risk of congenital anomalies. Which one of the following congenital anomalies are her babies at higher risk of developing?**

    A. Cataracts
    B. Foetal growth restriction
    C. Oligohydramnios
    D. Renal dysplasia
    E. Ventricular septal defects

7. **You are considering medical treatment for a 54-year-old woman with confirmed overactive bladder syndrome which has not responded to conservative measures.**

    Antimuscarinic therapy is contraindicated in which one of the following medical conditions?

    A. Anaemia
    B. Asthma
    C. Cataracts
    D. Hypothyroidism
    E. Ulcerative colitis

8. **Your medical students ask you about the use of foetal blood sampling in labour. Which one of the following is a contraindication to foetal blood sampling?**

    A. Antepartum haemorrhage
    B. Foetal tachycardia
    C. Immune thrombocytopaenic purpura
    D. Term breech
    E. Twin pregnancies

9. **You are reviewing a patient diagnosed with premature ovarian failure. She asks you what the recommended intake of calcium is. Which one of the following is correct?**

    A. 500 mg daily
    B. 600 mg daily
    C. 800 mg daily
    D. 1,000 mg daily
    E. 1,200 mg daily

10. **A 32-year-old woman presents with nausea and moderate abdominal pain. She is known to the assisted conception unit and was given human chorionic gonadotrophin (HCG) seven days ago. Ultrasound examination shows ascites and bilateral ovarian cysts which are 8–10 cm in size, with good blood flow. Blood investigations appear normal.**

    Which one of the following is the correct diagnosis?

    A. Early onset mild ovarian hyperstimulation syndrome (OHSS)
    B. Early onset moderate OHSS
    C. Late-onset mild OHSS
    D. Late-onset moderate OHSS
    E. Severe OHSS

11. **You are asked to review a 26-year-old primigravid woman in spontaneous labour with a continuing bradycardia. Examination findings are as follows:**

    Vertex 0/5 palpable per abdomen, cervix fully dilated, cephalic presentation at zero station and anterior fontanelle palpable with orbital ridges and nasal bridge felt anteriorly.

    Which one of the following is the most appropriate management?

    A. Category 1 emergency caesarean section
    B. Commence pushing
    C. Foetal blood sample
    D. Forceps delivery
    E. Ventouse delivery in the room

12. **A 27-year-old nulliparous woman presents with intermenstrual and post-coital bleeding. Cervical smear and biopsy confirm cervical cancer. She is keen on conservative management. Which one of the following dimensions of a tumour is suitable for cone biopsy?**

    A. 3 mm wide and 7 mm deep
    B. 5 mm wide and 3 mm deep
    C. 5 mm wide and 5 mm deep
    D. 6 mm wide and 3 mm deep
    E. 10 mm wide and 10 mm deep

13. **You are performing a category 1 emergency caesarean section in a woman with a confirmed placental abruption. Whilst delivering the placenta, you notice that her blood is not clotting. While waiting for the results of coagulation studies, you speak to the haematologist on call.**

    Which one of the following is your immediate management?

    A. Administer 2 L Hartmann's solution
    B. Administer 4 units type-specific whole blood
    C. Administer 6 units cryoprecipitate
    D. Administer 6 units FFP
    E. Request 4 units Rhesus-negative unmatched blood

14. **Which one of the following is not an autosomal dominant condition:**

    A. Cystic fibrosis
    B. Huntington's chorea
    C. Marfan's syndrome
    D. Muscular dystrophy
    E. Neurofibromatosis

15. **As regards recurrent first-trimester miscarriage (RCM) in a 22-year-old woman, which one of the following is correct?**

    A. Antiphospholipid syndrome is associated with preterm labour as well as RCM
    B. Antiphospholipid syndrome is seen in 5% of women with RCM
    C. Antithrombotic prophylaxis should be given to women with RCM
    D. Serial cervical length should be performed
    E. A woman who has had one miscarriage at six weeks, and two terminations of pregnancy at seven and nine weeks of gestation can be considered as to have RCM

16. **Upon reviewing the results of the quadruple screen for a 39-year-old woman in her first pregnancy, you find abnormally low levels of alpha-fetoprotein, unconjugated oestriol, and HCG. The inhibin A level is normal.**

    Which one of the following is the most likely diagnosis?

    A. Open neural tube defects
    B. Trisomy 13
    C. Trisomy 18
    D. Trisomy 21
    E. Turner's syndrome

17. **A 34-year-old primiparous woman is seen in an antenatal clinic wishing to discuss vaccination in pregnancy. Which one of the following vaccines can be administered in pregnancy?**

    A. Influenza
    B. Measles
    C. Mumps
    D. Rubella
    E. Varicella zoster

18. **A 42-year-old nulliparous solicitor and her partner come to see you with a two-year history of primary infertility. Investigations are normal. She would like to know whether ICSI or IVF with donor oocytes is her best form of management.**

    Donor oocytes should be considered in managing fertility problems associated with which one of the following conditions?

    A. Failed IVF
    B. Ovarian failure following chemotherapy or radiotherapy
    C. Premature ovarian failure
    D. Turner's syndrome
    E. Unilateral oophorectomy

19. **A 38-year-old woman presents in her second pregnancy at 32 weeks gestation with itching on her palms and soles. She is diagnosed to have obstetric cholestasis (OC). Which one of the following is a complication associated with OC?**

    A. Antepartum haemorrhage
    B. Foetal growth restriction
    C. Pre-eclampsia
    D. Preterm delivery
    E. Stillbirth, requiring delivery before 37 weeks gestation

20. **A 23-year-old primiparous woman is referred to antenatal clinic with a known diagnosis of polycystic ovary syndrome (PCOS). Which one of the following risks is associated with pregnancy and PCOS?**
    A. Foetal growth restriction
    B. Instrumental delivery
    C. Placenta praevia
    D. Pre-eclampsia
    E. Twin pregnancy

21. **A 32-year-old multiparous woman presents with contractions every five minutes at 31 weeks gestation each lasting for 10–15 seconds. Which one of the following is an evidence-based statement about tocolysis?**
    A. Atosiban does not offer any difference in tocolysis than beta-agonists
    B. Compared with beta-agonists, nifedipine is associated with improvement in neonatal outcome
    C. Tocolysis has no clear effect on perinatal or neonatal morbidity
    D. Tocolytic drugs do not improve outcome
    E. Tocolytic drugs reduce the proportion of births occurring up to seven days after beginning treatment

22. **A 32-year-old woman with pelvic pain is diagnosed to have endometriosis. She has been trying to conceive for over 18 months. Which one of the following is correct?**
    A. Laparoscopic surgical treatment improves the chances of pregnancy in women with minimal or mild endometriosis
    B. Medical therapy of endometriosis should be offered to women with minimal or mild endometriosis attempting to conceive
    C. Postoperative medical treatment with GnRH analogue is recommended in women with moderate or severe endometriosis who are trying to conceive, because it improves pregnancy rates
    D. Presence of endometriosis does not affect the chance of live birth with IVF
    E. Women with severe endometriosis undergoing IVF have a lower chance of pregnancy if IVF is preceded by several months of pituitary downregulation

23. **A 30-year-old primigravida woman comes to the antenatal clinic to discuss the results of her screening investigations which gave a risk of trisomy 21 of 1 in 200. Which of the following is true?**
    A. Amniocentesis is safe at 14 + 0 weeks gestation
    B. Cell culture following amniocentesis fails in 2% of cases
    C. Due to her risk, invasive testing should be offered
    D. The miscarriage rate of amniocentesis is around 3%
    E. The risk of severe sepsis following amniocentesis is <0.1%

24. **A 37-year-old woman presents in her first pregnancy, anxious about the risk of perineal tears given her mother's history of a forceps delivery and third-degree tear. Which one of the following is correct?**
    A. 1% of all perineal tears are third- or fourth-degree tears
    B. All women should be offered physiotherapy and pelvic floor exercises for 4–6 weeks after a fourth-degree tear
    C. Perineal tears are more likely in post-term deliveries
    D. Women who have abnormal endo-anal ultrasonography should be offered a prophylactic episiotomy in subsequent pregnancies
    E. Women who have had a third- or fourth-degree tear should be offered a prophylactic episiotomy in subsequent pregnancies

25. **At a journal club meeting, a paper based on comparative studies without randomization is discussed. What evidence level is this classified as?**
    A. 1A
    B. 2B
    C. 3
    D. 3C
    E. 4

26. **A 33-year-old woman consults you for contraception following her second delivery. She does not want oral medication and asks about the combined vaginal ring. Which one of the following is correct?**
    A. It contains ethinylestradiol and levonorgestrel
    B. It is changed every six months
    C. It is unaffected by enzyme-inducing drugs
    D. It should be kept refrigerated before use
    E. The risk of venous thromboembolism (VTE) is reduced when compared with combined oral contraception (COC)

27. **A 28-year-old woman undergoes a LLETZ procedure for CIN 3. Which one of the following is correct?**
    A. LLETZ excision should be at least 15 mm in depth
    B. Vaginal intercourse and tampons should be avoided for ten days after LLETZ
    C. Women should be warned that menstrual bleeding may be more sustained and heavier following LLETZ
    D. Women undergoing a LLETZ should be warned of an increased risk of infertility
    E. Women who have had a LLETZ procedure should be counselled on the increased risk of perinatal mortality in pregnancy

28. **A multiparous woman from an area with a known high prevalence of hepatitis B carriers status books at 22 weeks of pregnancy. Which one of the following is correct?**

    A. Hepatitis B specific immunoglobulins are sufficient for protecting her newborn against transmission

    B. She should have tests for hepatitis B antibodies first, and antigen tests if she is found to be antibody-positive

    C. She would be highly infectious if the hepatitis B surface antigen (HBsAg) is positive

    D. She would be of low infectivity if the hepatitis B 'e' antigen (HBeAg) is positive

    E. There is a chance of exacerbating her hepatitis B after the end of the pregnancy

29. **A 29-year-old woman presents with an intrauterine foetal death at 29 weeks. You are asked to prescribe mifepristone. What type of drug is this?**

    A. Glucocorticoid agonist

    B. Oestrogen antagonist

    C. Oxytocic agonist

    D. Progesterone antagonist

    E. Prostaglandin analogue

30. **A 32-year-old nulliparous woman presents with a six-month history of worsening vulval pain. She is diagnosed to have vulvodynia. What is your first-line treatment?**

    A. 1% lidocaine ointment

    B. 2% lidocaine ointment

    C. Amitriptyline, at the same dose as used for treating depression

    D. Clobetasone butyrate cream

    E. Gabapentin tablets

31. **A 27-year-old woman presents to clinic with a 4 cm simple unilateral ovarian cyst. She is worried about the risk of ovarian cancer, as her aunt died of ovarian cancer. Which one of the following is a risk factor for ovarian cancer?**

    A. Breastfeeding

    B. Hysterectomy

    C. Nulliparity

    D. Tubal ligation

    E. Use of the oral contraceptive pill

32. **A 19-year-old woman presents with hot sweats and tremor at 19 weeks gestation in her first pregnancy. She is noted to have thyroid enlargement and you suspect thyrotoxicosis. Which one of the following is correct?**

    A. Beta-agonists should be prescribed to control tachycardia

    B. Breastfeeding is contraindicated

    C. Diagnosis relies on a raised free T3, suppressed TSH level, and low free T4 level

    D. Fine needle biopsy is contraindicated in pregnancy

    E. Uncontrolled hyperthyroidism increases the risk of IUGR

33. **A 32-year-old multiparous woman is found to have a malignant breast lump in her first trimester of pregnancy. Which one of the following is correct?**

A. An echocardiogram should be performed in pregnancy for women who have had adjuvant chemotherapy with anthracyclines (e.g. doxorubicin)

B. Long-term survival of breast cancer is better in those women diagnosed in pregnancy

C. Tamoxifen is contraindicated in the first trimester of pregnancy only

D. Women can breastfeed while on tamoxifen

E. Women with breast cancer should be advised not to breastfeed from the affected breast

34. **A 37-year-old primiparous woman presents at 32 weeks gestation to discuss her birth plan. She is particularly concerned about the impact of an emergency caesarean section (CS) at full dilatation. Which one of the following is correct?**

A. CS at full dilatation with no attempt at operative vaginal delivery is associated with a higher risk of urinary and bowel complications when compared to CS at full dilatation after a failed instrumental delivery

B. The frequency of constipation at one year is higher with CS at full dilatation than with operative delivery

C. Neonatal asphyxia is 1.5 times more likely with CS at full dilatation than CS during the first stage of labour

D. Neonatal trauma is greater with an operative delivery than CS at full dilatation

E. There is an increase in neonatal sepsis with CS at full dilatation

35. **A 62-year-old woman was referred urgently to the outpatient hysteroscopy clinic with a history of postmenopausal bleeding for three days. Hysteroscopy showed a benign-looking endometrial polyp (approximately 2.5 cm in length) arising from the left lateral wall. Which one is the correct answer?**

A. Uterine curettage for removal of polyp

B. Conservative management

C. Endometrial ablation

D. Endometrial biopsy

E. Hysteroscopic resection of endometrial polyp and endometrial biopsy under general or local anaesthetic

36. **A 60-year-old woman presents with vault prolapse. In treating post-hysterectomy vaginal vault prolapse, the operation with the highest success rate is:**

A. Anterior vaginal repair

B. Iliococcygeous fixation

C. Posterior vaginal repair

D. Sacrocolpopexy

E. Sacrospinous fixation

37. **You review the MRI results of a 68-year-old nulliparous woman who is being staged for ovarian cancer. Results suggest the tumour involves both ovaries with microscopically confirmed peritoneal metastasis outside the pelvis with microscopic peritoneal metastasis beyond the pelvis (maximum size 2 cm). What stage of ovarian cancer does she have?**
    A. Stage 2C
    B. Stage 3A
    C. Stage 3B
    D. Stage 3C
    E. Stage 4

38. **A 32-year-old primiparous woman presents at 37 weeks gestation with breech presentation. Which one of the following is a cause of persistent breech presentation?**
    A. Grand multiparity
    B. Large-for-dates foetus
    C. Oligohydramnios
    D. Placental abruption
    E. Trisomy 21

39. **A 23-year-old primiparous woman with known depression attends your antenatal clinic. What impact can maternal depression have on the developing foetus?**
    A. Congenital heart defects
    B. Foetal tachycardia
    C. Higher risk of caesarean delivery
    D. Low birthweight
    E. Placental abruption

40. **A 20-year-old woman alleges vaginal and oral rape 48 hours ago. Which one of the following statements is correct with regard to providing aftercare?**
    A. Blood should be taken for HIV, syphilis, and hepatitis B and C serology at baseline and repeated after 12 weeks
    B. Hepatitis B immunoglobulin should routinely be offered
    C. HIV post-exposure prophylaxis after sexual exposure (PEPSE) should routinely be offered
    D. If emergency contraception (EC) is required, then hormonal emergency contraception is preferable over a post-coital copper IUD because of the increased risk of PID
    E. Prophylactic antibiotics covering chlamydia and gonorrhoea should routinely be offered

41. **A 27-year-old woman in her first pregnancy gives a 36-hour history of leaking clear fluid continuously. She is 31 weeks gestation with no abdominal pain or vaginal bleeding. Which one initial investigation would you request in the management of this woman?**

    A. Amniocentesis
    B. Biophysical profile
    C. Cardiotocography
    D. Transabdominal ultrasound assessment of cervical length
    E. Ultrasound assessment for growth

42. **You are reviewing a 22-year-old epileptic woman following a normal vaginal delivery three hours ago. She lives with her four-year-old son in a flat on the sixth floor.**

    Which one is the most important consideration during the post-partum period?

    A. The baby's nappies should be changed on the floor
    B. Breastfeeding should be avoided
    C. The neonate should be given 1 mg intramuscular vitamin K daily for the first week
    D. The patient can be discharged home with follow-up with her GP
    E. The risk of having a seizure in the first 24 hours after delivery is approximately 10%

43. **You receive the following result for a 25-year-old woman in her first pregnancy at 26 weeks: CMV-specific immunoglobulin M-positive; CMV-specific immunoglobulin G-negative.**

    Which one of the following describes the risk of vertical transmission to the foetus at this stage in pregnancy?

    A. 10%
    B. 20%
    C. 40%
    D. 60%
    E. 80%

44. **A 29-year-old nulliparous woman comes to see you in the clinic following a knife cone biopsy for stage 1A1 cervical cancer.**

    Which one is the most significant risk for this woman during pregnancy?

    A. Chorioamnionitis
    B. Infertility
    C. Low birthweight
    D. Placental abruption
    E. Premature rupture of membranes

45. A 24-year-old woman presents with sudden onset of itching, burning, and irritation of the vulva. She is fit and well. She suffers from eczema, and had an episode of hay fever recently. She has recently started a new relationship. Inspection reveals vesicles and weeping of the skin on both labial folds with oedema and crusting.

Which one is the most likely diagnosis in this patient?

A. Allergic dermatitis
B. Herpes infection
C. Irritant dermatitis
D. Lichen planus
E. Lichen simplex chronicus

46. You review a 26-year-old woman with mild hirsutism and oligomenorrhoea. The blood investigations suggest PCOS and ultrasound confirms a diagnosis of polycystic ovaries.

Which one of the following is a consequence of PCOS?

A. Intervals between menstruation of more than three months may be associated with endometrial hyperplasia
B. PCOS women who are oligomenorrhoeic do not need any further investigations
C. Risk of miscarriage in PCOS women is similar to that in the general population
D. There is an association with breast or ovarian cancer but no additional surveillance is required
E. There is an association with infertility but no additional assessment is required

47. A 34-year-old woman has been diagnosed with gestational trophoblastic neoplasia (GTN). Which one of the following is correct advice?

A. The cure rate for GTN is 89%
B. In patients with a FIGO (2000) score above 5, multiagent chemotherapy is indicated
C. IUCD contraception should be administered two weeks after surgical treatment
D. Single-agent chemotherapy advances the age of menopause by three years
E. There is a higher risk of thromboembolism with GTN

48. You review a 27-year-old woman with her partner following their first pregnancy, which resulted in a preterm delivery at 25 weeks gestation. Which one of the following infections can directly cause preterm labour?

A. E.coli urinary tract infection
B. HIV
C. Mycobacterium tuberculosis
D. Severe herpes genitalis with cervical lesions
E. Syphilis

49. You are reviewing a 37-year-old woman and her partner, who have consulted you following two first-trimester miscarriages.

Which one management plan would you recommend for this couple?

A. Anti-lupus coagulant should be checked

B. An elective cervical cerclage should be considered in her next pregnancy

C. Progesterone supplementation is recommended

D. Reassurance—no investigations are indicated

E. Serial cervical sonographic surveillance should take place in her next pregnancy

50. You are reviewing a 45-year-old woman who is booked for a total abdominal hysterectomy. She tells you that she suffered a wound breakdown after her skin stitches were removed after a CS seven years ago.

Which one suture type has longest absorbability time?

A. PDS

B. Polydioxanone

C. Polyglactin

D. Polyglycolic acid

E. Polypropylene

Extended Matching Questions

Options for Questions 1–5

For each of the following clinical scenarios, choose the most appropriate management option from the list provided. Each option may be used once, more than once, or not at all.

A. ARM
B. ARM, FSE, syntocinon augmentation
C. Category 1 CS
D. Category 2 CS
E. Category 3 CS
F. Category 4 CS
G. Continue pushing for a further one hour
H. Foetal blood sample
I. Forceps
J. FSE and FBS
K. Reassess, continue for pushing one hour, with fifteen-minute reviews
L. Stop CTG
M. Trial of forceps
N. Vacuum extraction

1. A 27-year-old primigravid woman presents to labour ward in spontaneous labour at term. Foetal assessment is reassuring and at vaginal examination, she is 9 cm dilated with a face presentation. The position is mento-posterior.

2. A 32-year-old primigravid woman has progressed well in spontaneous labour at term and has been pushing for one hour with no signs of an imminent delivery. At her last vaginal examination, the position was direct occipito-anterior.

3. A 32-year-old multiparous woman who has previously had a forceps delivery for failure to progress in the second stage was admitted to labour ward for an epidural. She has pushed for 30 minutes but is now exhausted. A vaginal examination demonstrates direct occipito-anterior position at spines, but there is little descent secondary to poor maternal effort.

4. A 29-year-old multiparous woman is admitted to labour ward at 6 cm dilatation at 32 weeks gestation. A CTG is commenced and demonstrates a baseline foetal heart rate of 140 bpm with deep variable decelerations to 60 bpm with slow recovery and normal variability. There is meconium staining of the liquor. The midwife has tried a change of maternal position for the past 90 minutes with no improvement in the trace.

5. A 19-year-old primigravid woman is admitted to the labour ward in early labour at 41 + 4 weeks gestation. She is 1 cm dilated and a CTG is commenced. This demonstrates a foetal baseline of 130 bpm, variability 5–15 bpm, accelerations, and no decelerations.

Options for Questions 6–10

For each of the following clinical scenarios, choose the most appropriate management option from the list provided. Each option may be used once, more than once, or not at all.

A. Blood transfusion
B. Diagnostic laparoscopy and proceed
C. Fluid resuscitation
D. Fluid resuscitation, and proceed to laparotomy

E. Hormone profile

F. Laparoscopic salpingotomy

G. Laparotomy and proceed

H. Methotrexate at dose of 50 mg/m²

I. Methotrexate at dose of 100 mg

J. Progesterone

K. Repeat HCG 24 hours

L. Repeat HCG 48 hours

M. Repeat TVUSS

N. TVUSS, serum HCG, chlamydia test

O. USS and serum HCG

6. A 26-year-old nulliparous woman attends the early pregnancy clinic at eight weeks of amenorrhoea with a positive home pregnancy test. She reports vaginal spotting and pain on intercourse.

7. A 32-year-old multiparous woman attends for an early reassurance scan. The uterus is empty and there is no sign of an extrauterine pregnancy. The serum HCG was initially 4,500 and 48 hours later was 5,000. She has had two previous CSs.

8. A 32-year-old multiparous woman attends for an early reassurance scan. The uterus is empty and the HCG is 950. She has had three laparotomies for Crohn's disease.

9. A 25-year-old woman in her second pregnancy at ten weeks of amenorrhoea attends casualty via ambulance after collapsing at home with abdominal pain. She is pale, clammy, has a distended abdomen and generalized abdominal guarding. Her urine pregnancy test is positive. She is a Jehovah's Witness.

10. A 29-year-old woman is diagnosed with an ectopic pregnancy. There is a 3 cm right-sided mass on USS with a visible foetal heartbeat and no free fluid in the pelvis. The HCG is static at 3,500. She wishes to avoid surgery.

Options for Questions 11–15

Select the most likely diagnosis that best matches the following description. Each option may be used once, more than once, or not at all.

A. Basal cell carcinoma

B. Candida

C. Condylomata

D. Dermatitis

E. Differentiated type VIN

F. Eczema

G. Lichen planus

H. Lichen sclerosus

I. Lichen simplex

J. Paget's disease

K. Psoriasis

L. Squamous cell carcinoma

M. Usual-type VIN

11. A 55-year-old woman presents with pruritus and an erythematous rash on the vulva. On examination the rash has a 'strawberries-and-cream' appearance with signs of lichenification. She has recently been diagnosed with breast adenocarcinoma.

12. A 61-year-old woman recently diagnosed with type 2 diabetes presents with a two-week history of vulval itching and soreness. On examination there is a clearly defined area of inflammation involving the perineum with satellite lesions on her mons pubis.

13. A 40-year-old woman presents with a two-month history of multiple red nodules on her vulva and dyspareunia. She is a smoker and has had previous 'treatment to the cervix' for 'an abnormal smear'.

14. A 75-year-old woman presents with a six-month history of severe vulval pruritus and pain, especially at night, which is preventing her from sleeping. On examination, the skin is atrophic with a 'cigarette paper' appearance and distorted anatomy.

15. A 28-year-old nulliparous woman presents with a history of worsening irritation around the vaginal introitus and increasing difficulty during intercourse. Her symptoms have not responded to topical steroids.

Options for Questions 16–20

For each of the following clinical scenarios, choose the most appropriate option. Each option may be used once, more than once, or not at all.

A. Abdominal ultrasound scan
B. Anterior colporrhaphy
C. Anticholinergics
D. Bulking agents
E. Colposuspension
F. Desmopressin
G. Detrusor myomectomy
H. Intravesical Botox injections
I. Intravesical hyaluronic acid
J. Pelvic and abdominal ultrasound scan
K. Pessary
L. Physiotherapy
M. Physiotherapy, bladder training
N. Standard cystometry
O. Tape procedure
P. Urodynamics

16. A 40-year-old multiparous woman was referred by her GP due to prolapse and mixed urinary incontinence. On examination she has a grade 1 cystocele and rectocele (pelvic organ prolapse quantification, POPQ). No stress incontinence is demonstrable. Her bladder diary is suggestive of frequency and urgency. Which one of the following is the most appropriate initial management option?

17. A 55-year-old woman has been diagnosed with interstitial cystitis. Oral therapy has been unhelpful. Which one is the next available management option?

18. A 60-year-old woman who underwent TVT-O two years ago has attended for follow-up with recurrent stress incontinence. Conservative management has failed and clinically, stress incontinence is demonstrable. She is now requesting further surgical treatment. Which one is the next management option?

19. A 49-year-old woman with three children born by vaginal delivery presents with leaking on exercise, coughing, and sneezing, with occasional urgency. She has tried pelvic floor exercises with little improvement in her symptoms and seeks definitive treatment. On examination there is minimal prolapse and urinalysis is clear. Which one is the next management option?

20. A 73-year-old woman presents with symptoms of urgency and urge incontinence. She states her abdomen feels more bloated and she cannot do the top button of her trousers up anymore. Urinalysis is clear. Which one is the next management option?

Options for Questions 21–25

For each of the following clinical scenarios, choose the most appropriate option. Each option may be used once, more than once, or not at all.

    A. Clomiphene citrate
    B. Diagnostic hysteroscopy
    C. Diagnostic hysteroscopy and diagnostic laparoscopy dye test
    D. Diagnostic laparoscopy and saline test
    E. Hysterosalpingogram
    F. Laparoscopy and methylene blue dye test
    G. Offer insertion of cervical suture in second trimester
    H. Offer insertion of prophylactic cervical suture in first trimester
    I. Offer insertion of prophylactic suture in first trimester
    J. Reassurance
    K. Saline hysteroscopy
    L. Ultrasound cervical length assessment during first and second trimesters
    M. Vaginal progesterone suppositories from 13 weeks onwards

21. A 35-year-old woman who has had two previous painless miscarriages in the second trimester had normal baseline investigations. She is concerned about the risk of preterm labour.

22. A 30-year-old multiparous woman who has had two caesarean sections is being investigated for secondary infertility. She has a history of pelvic infection in the past.

23. A 38-year-old nulliparous woman with primary infertility of five years' duration has a history of irregular painful heavy periods and deep dyspareunia.

24. A 29-year-old multiparous woman with a BMI of 32 with mid-luteal progesterone of 8 nmol/L. She has no relevant gynaecology history.

25. A 38-year-old nulliparous woman with a BMI of 35 with mid-luteal phase progesterone of 36 nmol/L and regular cycles.

Options for Questions 26–30

For each of the following clinical scenarios, choose the most appropriate option. Each option may be used once, more than once, or not at all.

    A. Aspirin and low molecular weight heparin
    B. Assisted conception treatment
    C. Cervical length assessment
    D. Clindamycin cream
    E. Folic acid
    F. High-dose steroids
    G. Low-dose aspirin
    H. Metformin
    I. Partner's white cell infusion
    J. Pre-implantation genetic diagnosis
    K. Reassurance
    L. Uterine reconstructive surgery
    M. Weight management

26. A 30-year-old woman with three first-trimester pregnancy losses and normal BMI has normal investigation results for recurrent miscarriage.
27. A 37-year-old woman with four first-trimester pregnancy losses has thrombophilia screening test reported positive on two separate occasions.
28. A 30-year-old nulliparous woman has a history of recurrent miscarriage with a BMI 40 and normal thrombophilia screening.
29. A 25-year-old woman who has had one spontaneous pregnancy loss during the second trimester.
30. A 30-year-old woman with a history of recurrent miscarriage and a normal BMI is diagnosed with an arcuate uterus.

Options for Questions 31–35

You are in the antenatal clinic. Choose the best course of management for each scenario. Each option may be used once, more than once, or not at all.

A. Admit at 38 weeks until delivery
B. Admit until delivery
C. Caesarean section and sterilization
D. Discharge to midwife-led care
E. ECV at 37–38 weeks
F. Elective LSCS
G. Emergency LSCS
H. Offer vaginal breech delivery
I. Reassure
J. Steroids, offer vaginal breech delivery
K. Ultrasound growth scan
L. Ultrasound scan for placental site

31. A 24-year-old woman with four previous normal vaginal deliveries is referred in by the midwife for confirmation of presentation at 36 weeks. You see from the notes that on abdominal palpation the baby was felt to be breech initially, then cephalic yesterday. The woman reports many foetal movements and that the baby is a 'wriggler'. Today the presentation is breech, and is not engaged.
32. A 32-year-old woman is referred in at 36 weeks with a continuing breech presentation. She has had one previous normal delivery. She has been seen in the community throughout and she is keen on a home birth. On examination today, the baby's presentation is breech.
33. You see a grand multiparous woman (four vaginal deliveries followed by two caesarean sections) who has now reached 40 + 12 weeks gestation. She has had a breech presentation throughout her pregnancy. She is keen on a vaginal birth should labour occur spontaneously but there are no signs of labour. A recent ultrasound scan suggests an estimated foetal weight of 3.9 kg.
34. A midwife has referred a 30-year-old primigravid woman to see you after her 24-week appointment. The woman is very concerned as the baby's presentation was breech on her 20-week scan.
35. You see a 27-year-old, 32-week-pregnant woman in clinic with breech presentation. She is complaining of severe intermittent abdominal pain. You refer her to triage for assessment and your junior calls to ask for advice as she is found to be 4 cm dilated and is having two uterine contractions every 10 minutes. The membranes ruptured during examination and she is draining clear liquor.

Options for Questions 36–40

From the following list of statistical terms, choose the most appropriate for each of the descriptions provided. Each option may be used once, more than once, or not at all.

A. Accuracy
B. False-negative rate
C. False-positive rate
D. Likelihood ratio
E. Negative predictive value
F. Odds ratio
G. Positive predictive value
H. Screen-positive rate
I. Sensitivity
J. Specificity
K. True positive rate

36. The ability of a screening test to identify unaffected individuals.
37. The likelihood that an individual screened positive for the condition actually has the disease.
38. The proportion of individuals screened positive who do not actually have the condition.
39. The proportion of the screened population who have a positive result.
40. The ability of a test to identify affected individuals.

Options for Questions 41–45

Match each of the following case scenarios with the most appropriate treatment from the list provided. Each option may be used once, more than once, or not at all.

A. Abdominal sacropexy
B. Colpocleisis
C. Paravaginal repair
D. Pelvic floor exercises
E. Posterior vaginal wall repair
F. Posterior vaginal wall repair with mesh
G. Ring pessary
H. Sacrospinous vault fixation
I. Shelf pessary
J. Traditional anterior repair
K. Uterosacral ligament suspension

41. A 48-year-old woman presents with 'something coming down' for the past six months. She has previously had a vaginal hysterectomy for heavy periods. She is sexually active and denies any bladder or bowel symptoms. On examination, she has stage 3 vault prolapse and stage 1 anterior prolapse.
42. A 60-year-old woman presents with 'something coming down' and difficulty emptying her bowels. She has had a vaginal hysterectomy and posterior repair five years ago and was well for the first two years post-operation. She does not report any urinary symptoms. She is not sexually active. Examination reveals a stage 2 posterior wall prolapse, stage 1 vault descent, and a well-supported anterior vaginal wall.
43. A 58-year-old sexually active woman presents with a sensation of a bulge 'down below' and difficulty sometimes initiating urinary voiding. On examination she has stage 2 anterior

compartment prolapse. The vault is well supported, as is the posterior vaginal wall. She is having to spend increasing amounts of time caring for her invalid child and is keen on a definitive treatment as soon as possible.

44. A 77-year-old healthy woman presents with symptoms suggestive of prolapse. She has struggled for many years with this problem, and indeed has undergone a number of surgeries, including vaginal hysterectomy, to treat prolapse in all three compartments. The problem has recurred and examination shows a recurrence of stage 2–3 prolapse. Pessaries have previously been poorly tolerated. She is not sexually active.

45. A 54-year-old woman who had has three children presents with a sensation of a bulge 'down below' with no urinary or bowel symptoms. On examination, she has stage 2 anterior compartment prolapse. There is no uterine descent and the posterior vaginal wall is well supported.

Options for Questions 46–50

Match the employer or their job description with the following personnel. Each option may be used once, more than once, or not at all.

- A. Consultant or senior colleague
- B. Could change the decision
- C. Could not change the decision
- D. Court of protection
- E. Crown office
- F. Deputy
- G. Lasting power of attorney
- H. Office of the public guardian
- I. Procurator fiscal/coroner

46. An official appointed by the court of protection.

47. An ability to choose one or more people to make decisions about health or finance.

48. Information which is available to make decisions to appoint someone to get help.

49. Personnel who make or help to make decisions for people on their health, finance, or welfare.

50. Government official working to inquire all reported deaths.

Single Best Answers

1. D. Pre-eclampsia

Smoking during pregnancy is associated with an increased incidence of miscarriage, preterm delivery, placental abruption, and placenta praevia. Maternal smoking has been associated with a reduced incidence of pre-eclampsia in women aged 30 years and under with no history of hypertension. Maternal smoking and especially passive smoking is also associated with increased risk of Sudden infant death syndrome (SIDS) and many other problems related to weaker lungs.

CDC. Smoking during pregnancy: smoking and tobacco use; 2022.

Eastham R, Gosakan R. Smoking and smoking cessation in pregnancy. *TOG* 2010;12:103–9.

2. B. Central nervous system changes

The higher the dose of radiation exposure, the more severe the effects on pregnancy. Effects include lethal effects (miscarriage), reduced cell division (foetal growth restriction), CNS changes, and foetal malformations. The commonest teratogenic effects of exposure to high-dose radiation are CNS changes—the risk of microcephaly and mental retardation begins at ten weeks gestation. The risk of developing childhood cancer after a VQ scan or CT is slightly higher with VQ scan. This risk is an extra one case for every 34,000 VQ scans performed.

Eskander OS, Eckford SD, Watkinson T. Safety of diagnostic imaging in pregnancy. Part 1: X-ray, nuclear medicine investigation, CT and contrast media. *TOG* 2010;12:71–8.

NHS. Investigation of suspected Pulmonary Embolism (PE) in pregnancy. Available at: https://www.hey. nhs.uk/patient-leaflet/investigation-of-suspected-pulmonary-embolism

3. E. Warfarin

Women who are taking liver enzyme-inducing drugs such as rifampicin and phenytoin should be offered alternative EC to the levonorgestrel pill due to the reduction in the efficacy of the pill. Women on warfarin should be informed that the anticoagulant effect can be altered and an INR test should be performed within 3–4 days of administering levonorgestrel.

Bhathena R, Guillebaud J. Postcoital contraception. *TOG* 2011;13:29–34.

4. B. Administer 5 mg folic acid until the end of the pregnancy

Anti-epileptic medication should be continued unless the woman has been seizure-free for a minimum of two years. Major congenital malformations are more likely with sodium valproate and carbamazepine than lamotrigine. The use of lamotrigine during pregnancy has not been associated with an increased risk of neural tube defects; however, the recommendation regarding higher doses of folic acid supplementation is often, but not always, broadened to include women taking any anticonvulsant, including lamotrigine. Folic acid 5 mg should be commenced at least three months before conception and till the beginning of second trimester. Vitamin K 10–20 mg oral should be prescribed from 36 weeks' gestation.

Nelson-Piercy C. *Handbook of obstetric medicine*, 5th ed. New York: Informa Healthcare; 2015.

NHS. Pregnancy, breastfeeding and fertility while taking lamotrigine. Available at: https://www.nhs.uk

5. A. Early menarche

Risk factors for dysmenorrhoea include early menarche, nulliparity, and a positive family history of dysmenorrhoea. Several studies suggest smoking is also a risk factor.

Wallace S, Keightley A, Gie C. Dysmenorrhoea. *TOG* 2010;12:149–54.

6. E. Ventricular septal defects

The congenital anomaly rate in monochorionic twins is three to four times higher than that of dichorionic twins or singleton pregnancies. Among monochorionic twins there are increased risks of cardiovascular and central nervous system malformations.

Devaseelan P, Ong S. Twin pregnancy: controversies in management. *TOG* 2010;12:179–85.

NICE: Twins and Triplet Pregnancy CG 137; 4 September 2019.

7. E. Ulcerative colitis

Absolute contraindications to antimuscarinics therapy include myasthenia gravis, ulcerative colitis, and glaucoma. Caution should be taken when prescribing antimuscarinics to hypothyroid patients.

Abboudi H, Fynes M, Doumouchtsis S. Contemporary therapy for the overactive bladder *TOG* 2011;13:98–106.

8. C. Immune thrombocytopaenic purpura

Foetal blood samples do not provide accurate results in immune thrombocytopaenic purpura and therefore should be avoided.

NICE Pathway. Fetal blood sampling; 2014

NICE. Intrapartum care for healthy women and babies, CG190 (updated 14 December 2022).

9. E. 1,200 mg daily

Menopausal women are at risk of osteoporosis and osteopenia. The recommended intake of calcium is 1,200 mg daily; for vitamin D it is 600–800 IU daily. HRT and weight-bearing exercises should also be considered to maintain bone mass.

Tong I. Non-pharmacological treatment of postmenopausal symptoms. *TOG* 2013;15:19–25.

NICE: Diagnosis and management of menopause, NG23 (last updated 5 December 2019).

10. B. Early-onset moderate OHSS

Early onset OHSS occurs within nine days of administering HCG and tends to be less severe than late OHSS. Mild OHSS presents with abdominal bloating, mild abdominal pain, and ovaries which are less than 8 cm in size. Moderate OHSS presents with moderate pain, nausea, vomiting, and ultrasound evidence of ascites, with ovaries 8–12 cm in size.

NICE. Fertility problems. Assessment and treatment, CG156; 2017.

Prakash A, Mathur R. Ovarian hyperstimulation syndrome. *TOG* 2013;15:31–5.

RCOG. Ovarian hyperstimulation syndrome (OHSS) patient information leaflet | RCOG

11. A. Category 1 emergency CS

This is a brow presentation, with the largest diameter presenting being mentovertical (13.5–14 cm). With a continuing bradycardia, category 1 emergency CS is the most appropriate management.

RCOG. StratOG: Management of normal labour and delivery: mechanisms of normal labour and delivery.

12. D. 6 mm wide and 3 mm deep

Women with FIGO stage 1A1 disease (squamous cell carcinoma of the cervix invading to a depth of 3 mm and width of <7 mm wide) can be treated with knife or laser cone biopsy alone, as long as there is no lympho-vascular space invasion.

Ellis P, Mould T. Fertility-saving treatment in gynaecological oncology. *TOG* 2009;11:239–44.

13. C. Administer six units of cryoprecipitate

When a major placental abruption develops, disseminated intravascular coagulation can quickly develop. Whilst waiting for coagulation studies and a platelet count, the advice of a haematologist should be sought. Up to four units of FFP and ten units of cryoprecipitate may be given whilst waiting for the results of the coagulation studies.

RCOG Green-top Guideline 63. Antepartum haemorrhage; November 2011.

14. A. Cystic fibrosis

Autosomal dominant conditions are ones that are expressed in heterozygotes (i.e. affected individuals need to carry only one copy of the mutated gene). They affect males and females in equal proportions. The chance of an affected individual passing the condition on to his or her offspring is 50%. Huntington's chorea is an example of an autosomal dominant condition. Cystic fibrosis is an example of an autosomal recessive condition. Marfan syndrome is an example of an autosomal dominant condition.

StratOG.net. Genetic disorders. RCOG online training resource

15. A. Antiphospholipid syndrome is associated with preterm labour and RCM as well

Recurrent miscarriage (RCM) is defined as having three consecutive miscarriages. However, most recent guidance recommends that, 'the new approach would be to see women offered information and guidance to support future pregnancies after one miscarriage, an appointment at a miscarriage clinic for initial investigations after two miscarriages, and a full series of evidence-based investigations and care—as described in this guideline—after three miscarriages'.

Antiphospholipid syndrome is seen in 15% of women with recurrent miscarriage. Antithrombotic prophylaxis should be given to women with antiphospholipid syndrome. No benefit is seen by performing serial cervical length measurements.

RCOG. New draft guideline outlines best practice for treating recurrent miscarriage; 2021.

16. C. Trisomy 18

The quadruple test involves measuring maternal serum levels of alpha-fetoprotein, HCG, unconjugated oestriol, and inhibin A. This has an 80% sensitivity rate and 7% false-positive rate for the detection of trisomy 21. It can also be used to detect other chromosomal and structural abnormalities. In open neural tube defects, alpha-fetoprotein levels are raised. In cases of trisomy 21, HCG and inhibin A levels are raised.

Lakhi N, Govind A, Moretti M, Jones J. Maternal serum analytes as markers of adverse obstetric outcome. *TOG* 2012;14:267–73.

17. A. Influenza

All live, attenuated vaccines are contraindicated in pregnancy. These include the MMR (measles, mumps, and rubella) and varicella zoster vaccines. The influenza and pneumococcus vaccines contain killed but previously virulent micro-organisms.

Centers for Disease Control and Prevention. Guidelines for vaccinating pregnant women; May 2008 (updated July 2012).

NHS. Vaccinations in pregnancy; 2022. Available at: https://www.nhs.uk/pregnancy/keeping-well/vaccinations

18. B. Ovarian failure following chemotherapy or radiotherapy

Advancing age after 40 reduces the success rate of IVF significantly with a much higher rate of spontaneous miscarriage rates. However, young donor oocytes fertilized with partner semen samples improve implantation rates significantly, hence a much higher pregnancy rate. This is the reason why many IVF centres in Europe offer this programme to older mothers. Women with ovarian failure can be managed through the same programme, provided they have a uterus which is hormonally primed to make it receptive to implantation.

NICE Clinical Guideline 156. Fertility; 2013.

19. D. Preterm delivery

OC typically presents without a rash, but with pruritus in the palms and soles of the feet, associated with abnormal liver function tests and bile acid levels. It is associated with the increased risks of preterm birth, especially iatrogenic, and amniotic fluid meconium. Ultrasound scans to monitor foetal growth, foetal Doppler's, and cardiotocography are not sensitive predictors of intrauterine foetal deaths. The widely adopted practice of offering delivery at 37 weeks gestation, or at diagnosis if this is after 37 weeks gestation, is not evidence-based. It is generally advised as there are no reliable predictors of stillbirths.

Nelson-Piercy C. *Handbook of obstetric medicine*, 5th ed. New York: Informa Healthcare; 2015.

RCOG Green-top Guideline 43. Obstetric cholestasis; April 2011.

20. D. Pre-eclampsia

Pregnancy in known PCOS women is associated with significantly higher risk for miscarriage, developing gestational diabetes, and hypertensive problems during pregnancy. It is recommended to have an OGTT before 20 weeks of gestation and antenatal care with specialist.

RCOG Green-top Guideline 33. Long-term consequences of polycystic ovary syndrome; 2014.

21. B. Compared with beta-agonists, nifedipine is associated with improvement in neonatal outcome

Tocolytic drugs reduce the chance of delivery within seven days, but there is no clear evidence that it affects perinatal mortality or serious neonatal morbidity. Tocolysis should be used for gaining time to complete the course of steroids and in-utero transfer. Beta-agonists have a higher adverse effect profile than nifedipine but neonatal outcome has not been shown to be improved.

NICE. Preterm labour and birth, NG25 (updated 2022)

22. A. Laparoscopic surgical treatment improves the chances of pregnancy in women with minimal or mild endometriosis

Medical hormonal treatment of endometriosis does not enhance fertility in minimal or mild endometriosis; the evidence for moderate or severe endometriosis is lacking. Laparoscopic ablation of endometriosis and adhesiolysis is associated with a higher chance of pregnancy than diagnostic laparoscopy in women with minimal or mild endometriosis who wish to conceive. Meta-analysis shows that IVF success rates are lower in women with endometriosis than in women with tubal disease. Postoperative medical treatment with danazol or GnRH analogue does not improve the chances of conception. Women with endometriosis have a higher IVF pregnancy rate if they receive downregulation with GnRH analogue for at least three months prior to the start of IVF.

ESHRE: ESHRE Guideline for the diagnosis and treatment of endometriosis. *Hum Reprod* 2005;20(10):2698–704.

ESHRE Guideline for the Diagnosis and Treatment of Endometriosis (updated in 2007).

NICE. Fertility problems: assessment and treatment, CG156; 2017 (updated).

Sallam HN, Garcia-Velasco JA, Dias S, Arici A, Abou-Setta AM. Long-term pituitary down-regulation before *in vitro* fertilization (IVF) for women with endometriosis. *Cochrane Database Syst Rev* 2006;1:CD004635.

23. E. The risk of severe sepsis following amniocentesis is <0.1%

This procedure should be carried out using an aseptic technique. Multiple attempts increase the risk of delayed rupture of membranes. Prophylactic antibiotics do not reduce risk of infection. Miscarriage rate following amniocentesis is <1% in experienced hands (0.2%-0.3%)

RCOG Green-top Guideline 8. Amniocentesis and chorionic villus sampling; 2010.

RCOG Consent Advice 6. Amniocentesis; 2006

Stenhouse EJ, et al. First-trimester combined ultrasound and biochemical screening for Down syndrome in routine clinical practice. *Prenat Diagn* 2004;24(10):774–80.

24. A. 1% of all perineal tears are third or fourth-degree tears

Although birthweight >4 kg is a risk factor for perineal tears, gestation alone is not a risk factor. All women should be offered physiotherapy and pelvic floor exercises for 6–12 weeks after sustaining a third- or fourth-degree tear. There is no evidence to support a prophylactic episiotomy in subsequent pregnancies following a third- or fourth-degree tear. Women who are symptomatic or who have abnormal endo-anal ultrasonography and/or manometry should have the option of an elective CS.

RCOG Green-top Guideline 29. The management of third- and fourth-degree perineal tears; 2007.

25. C. level of evidence 3

- 1A evidence is defined as evidence obtained from meta-analysis of randomized controlled trials.
- 1B evidence is that obtained from at least one randomized controlled trial.
- 2A is evidence obtained from at least one well-designed controlled study without randomization.
- 2B is evidence obtained from at least one other type of well-designed quasi-experimental study.
- Level 3 is evidence obtained from well-designed non-experimental descriptive studies such as comparative studies, correlation studies, and case studies. There is no 3C level in any classification.

- Level 4 evidence is obtained from expert committee reports or opinions and/or the clinical experience of respected authorities.

Oxford Centre for Evidence-based Medicine. Level of evidence; 2009.

26. D. It should be kept refrigerated before use

The combined vaginal ring (CVR) releases EE and etonogestrel at daily rates of 15 µg and 20 µg, respectively. The CVR is left in the vagina continuously for 21 days. After a ring-free interval of seven days to induce a withdrawal bleed, a new ring is inserted. Enzyme-inducing drugs increase the metabolism of oestrogens and progestogens, which may in turn reduce the contraceptive efficacy of all combined hormonal contraceptive methods (CHC) irrespective of the mode of delivery. The relative risk of venous thromboembolism (VTE) associated with CVR use compared with other combined methods is not known. In a study comparing haemostatic variables in CVR and COC users, the activity of antithrombin, protein C, and factor VII was higher in CVR users. The clinical significance of these coagulatory changes is unknown. Advice given about thrombosis risk with the CVR is therefore generally based on COC data.

The CVR must be stored in a pharmaceutical refrigerator at a temperature of 2–8°C until the point of dispensing to the patient. The total shelf life is 40 months; 36 months under refrigeration, and 4 months after dispensing. The storage requirements for the CVR may limit its acceptability in clinical practice.

Faculty of Sexual & Reproductive Health (FSRH), Clinical Effectiveness Unit (CEU). UK medical eligibility criteria (UKMEC): summary sheets; 2016 UKMEC April 2016 Summary Sheet (amended September 2019)—Faculty of Sexual and Reproductive Healthcare (fsrh.org).

Faculty of Sexual & Reproductive Health (FSRH). New product review: NuvaRing; 2009.

NICE. Scenario. Combined vaginal ring (last revised in September 2022) Scenario: [Combined contraceptive vaginal ring; management; contraception, combined hormonal methods; CKS; NICE.

Faculty of Sexual & Reproductive Health (FSRH), Clinical Effectiveness Unit (CEU). Clinical Guidance. Combined hormonal contraception; amended November 2020.

FSRH Clinical Guideline: combined hormonal contraception (January 2019, amended November 2020).

27. C. Women should be warned that menstrual bleeding may be more sustained and heavier following LLETZ

Meta-analyses of long-term observational data suggest that deep LLETZ treatment increases the risk of preterm delivery but not the risk of perinatal mortality or infertility. A minimum of three weeks is recommended before considering protected intercourse. In 19–48% of cases, menstrual bleeding may be more sustained or heavier. LLETZ excision should be at least 10 mm in depth.

NHS Cervical Screening Programme Guideline 20. *Colposcopy and programme management*, 2nd ed. NHSCSP; 2010.

28. E.
There is a chance of exacerbating her hepatitis B after the end of the pregnancy

The effect of pregnancy on replication of HBV and the effect of antiviral treatment on the immune system is poorly understood. Despite adopting combined immunization programmes, 5–10% of babies are born with HBV infection in hepatitis B e antigen positive pregnant women. Although HBV infection is well tolerated during pregnancy, severe hepatitis and hepatic failure, induced by perinatal hepatic flare reactions, still occur and can have an unfavourable outcome.

British Association for Sexual Health and HIV (BASSH). United Kingdom National Guidelines on the Management of Viral Hepatitis A, B, and C. Management of hepatitis B in pregnancy; 2008.

2017 interim update of the 2015 BASHH National Guidelines for the Management of the Viral Hepatitides (updated in 2018).

29. D. Progesterone antagonist

Mifepristone is a synthetic steroid with anti-progesterone activity. It competitively blocks progesterone and glucocorticoid receptors, stimulating prostaglandin production. Misoprostol is a prostaglandin analogue.

Nzewi C, Araklitis G, Narvekar N. The use of mifepristone and misoprostol in the management of late intrauterine fetal death. *TOG* 2014;16:233–8.

RCOG Green-top Guideline 55. Late intrauterine fetal death and stillbirth; 2011.

30. B. 2% lidocaine ointment

Medical treatment includes topical, intralesional, and oral medication. 2% or 5% lidocaine ointment/gel is known to improve symptoms when applied overnight as well as prior to intercourse. This is initial therapy. Tricyclic antidepressants can be prescribed at doses lower than that for depression, followed by anticonvulsants such as gabapentin.

Nagandla K, Sivalingam N. Vulvodynia: integrating current knowledge into clinical practice. *TOG* 2014;16:259–67.

31. C. Nulliparity

The risk of ovarian cancer is reduced in women who have had a pregnancy, had used the oral contraceptive pill, breastfed, and undergone tubal ligation or hysterectomy.

Gaughan EMG, Walsh TA. Risk-reducing surgery for women at high risk of epithelial ovarian cancer. *TOG* 2014;16:185–91.

32. E. Uncontrolled hyperthyroidism increases the risk of IUGR

Results suggestive of thyrotoxicosis include a raised free T3 level, suppressed TSH level, and a raised or normal free T4 level. Fine needle biopsy can be considered to exclude malignancy, but radioactive treatment or investigation should be avoided. Beta-blockers are used to control tachycardia or a thyrotoxic crisis. Uncontrolled hyperthyroidism increases the risk of IUGR. Breastfeeding is not contraindicated.

Nelson-Piercy C. *Handbook of obstetric medicine*, 5th ed. New York: Informa Healthcare; 2015.

33. A. An echocardiogram should be performed in pregnancy for women who have had adjuvant chemotherapy with anthracyclines (e.g. doxorubicin)

Tamoxifen is associated with foetal abnormalities and is therefore contraindicated in pregnancy. Women should be advised to delay conception for at least three months following treatment with tamoxifen as it has a long half-life. Most women are advised to wait for two years following treatment as the risk of recurrence is highest for the first three years following diagnosis. It is unknown whether tamoxifen is transmitted into breast milk, and thus women should be advised not to breastfeed while on tamoxifen. The same advice applies to herceptin. Current evidence suggests that long-term survival is unaffected by pregnancy. In the past, women were advised against pregnancy as many breast cancers are oestrogen-positive; however, several case-controlled studies demonstrate no difference in outcome. Anthracycline can cause a dose-dependent cumulative left ventricle dysfunction which can lead to cardiomyopathy; therefore an echocardiogram is important. In a woman who has completed treatment, there is no evidence to suggest that breastfeeding is related to a poorer outcome. Lactation is unlikely in the affected breast following surgery, and radiotherapy can cause fibrosis. Given the many advantages of breastfeeding, women should be encouraged to do so when possible.

RCOG Green-top Guideline 12. Pregnancy and breast cancer; 2011.

34. D. Neonatal trauma is greater with an operative delivery than CS at full dilatation

Studies suggest there is no significant difference in urinary or bowel complications following an attempt at operative vaginal delivery prior to CS when compared to immediate CS. Neonatal trauma is greater with an operative delivery than CS at full dilatation. The frequency of constipation is higher at one year following an operative delivery than CS at full dilatation.

Vousden N, et al. CS at full dilatation: incidence, impact and current management. *TOG* 2014;16:199–205.

35. E. Hysteroscopic resection of endometrial polyp and endometrial biopsy under general or local anaesthetic

Given the size of the polyp and the clinical presentation, it is best to resect the polyp under direct vision.

Annan J, et al. The management of endometrial polyps in the 21st century. *TOG* 2012;14(1) 33–8.

36. D. Sacrocolpopexy

Vaginal repair is inadequate and may shorten the vagina resulting in dyspareunia. Sacrospinous fixation may have lower postoperative morbidity; however, it has a higher failure rate. Iliococcygeous fixation is not routinely recommended.

RCOG Green-top Guideline 46. The management of post-hysterectomy vaginal vault prolapse; 2007.

37. C. Stage 3B

FIGO staging for ovarian cancer is as follows:

Stage 1: Tumour is confined to one or both ovaries.

1A: Only one ovary is affected by the tumour; the ovary capsule is intact.

1B: Both ovaries are affected by the tumour; the ovary capsule is intact.

1C: The tumour is limited to one or both ovaries, with any of the following: the ovary capsule is ruptured; the tumour is detected on the ovary surface; or positive malignant cells are detected in the ascites or peritoneal washings.

Stage 2: Tumour involves one or both ovaries and has extended into the pelvis.

2A: The tumour has extended to or been implanted in the uterus, the fallopian tubes, or both.

2B: The tumour has extended to another organ in the pelvis.

2C: Tumours are as defined in 2A and 2B, and malignant cells are detected in the ascites or peritoneal washings.

Stage 3: The tumour involves one or both ovaries with microscopically confirmed peritoneal metastasis outside the pelvis and/or regional lymph node metastasis, including liver capsule metastasis.

3A: Microscopic peritoneal metastasis beyond the pelvis.

3B: Microscopic peritoneal metastasis beyond the pelvis 2 cm or less.

3C: Microscopic peritoneal metastasis beyond the pelvis more than 2 cm in greatest dimension and/or regional lymph nodes metastasis.

Stage 4: Distant metastasis beyond the peritoneal cavity and liver parenchymal metastasis, Endometriod tumours and mucinous cystadenocarcinomas are subtypes of epithelial tumours, which are the most common subtypes of ovarian carcinoma.

FIGO. Ovarian cancer staging; 2014.

Reproduced from *International Journal of Gynecology & Obstetrics*, 124,1, Part J, 'Staging classification for cancer of the ovary, fallopian tube, and peritoneum', pp. 1–5, Copyright (2014), with permission from Elsevier and FIGO International Federation of Gynecology and Obstetrics.

38. C. Oligohydramnios

Causes of persistent breech presentation may be categorized as *foetal, uterine,* or *uterine anomaly*.

Foetal: foetal structural anomaly (e.g. hydrocephalus), multiple pregnancy, prematurity.

Uterine: abnormal liquor volume (oligohydramanios and polyhydramnios), low placental position.

Uterine anomaly: fibroids—intramural or submucous, *not* pedunculated, uterine septation, unicornuate, bicornuate uterus, multiparity.

RCOG Green-top Guideline 20a: External cephalic version and reducing the incidence of breech presentation; 2006.

RCOG Green-top Guideline 20b: Management of breech presentation; 2006.

39. D. Low birthweight

Maternal depression can adversely affect the developing foetus. Studies suggest an association with preterm birth, low birthweight, smaller head circumference, and low Apgar scores.

Chambers CD, et al. Selective serotonin-reuptake inhibitors and risk of persistent pulmonary hypertension of the newborn. *N Engl J Med* 2006;354:579–87.

Conlon O, Lynch J. Maternal depression: risk factors and treatment options during pregnancy. *TOG* 2008;10:151–5.

Kieler H, et al. Selective serotonin reuptake inhibitors during pregnancy and risk of persistent pulmonary hypertension in the newborn: population-based cohort study from the five Nordic countries. *BMJ* 2012;12;344:d8012.

40. A. Blood should be taken for HIV, syphilis, and hepatitis B and C serology at baseline and repeated after 12 weeks

This is the usual recommended follow-up schedule for BBV and syphilis serology, taking account of the usual incubation periods. Vaccination against hepatitis B should be offered if the victim is not known to be immune. Hepatitis B immunoglobulin is not routinely recommended, but should be considered after a known infectious contact or if the assailant is strongly suspected to have hepatitis B. The decision to give HIV PEPSE is based on an assessment of a range of HIV risk factors as outlined by the British Association of Sexual Health & HIV (BASHH) and the British HIV Association (BHIVA); see references for further details.

It is not a routine requirement after rape to offer HIV PEPSE, because of the side-effect profile and a lack of conclusive data about its efficacy and long-term toxicity. Prophylaxis against STIs can be offered as part of immediate medical aftercare post-sexual assault, but it is not recommended as routine practice. The advantages have to be weighed against the disadvantages. A copper IUD is the most effective method of post-coital contraception, which should be discussed with and offered to all women after unprotected sex. Prophylactic antibiotics may be advisable to minimize the risk of PID.

British Association of Sexual Health & HIV (BASHH). UK national guidelines on the management of adult and adolescent complainants of sexual assault; 2011/2012.

British Association of Sexual Health & HIV (BASHH). UK national guideline for the use of post-exposure prophylaxis for HIV following sexual exposure; 2011.

41. C. Cardiotocography

First-line investigations of PPROM usually include maternal observations, urine dipstick and cardiotocography, and blood investigations to exclude chorioamnionitis. The true and false-positive rates for abnormal biophysical profile in predicting chorioamnionitis is 30–80% and 2–9%, respectively. Foetal tachycardia has 20–40% sensitivity with a false-positive rate of around 3%. Transvaginal ultrasound is not contraindicated in the assessment of cervical length in PPROM, as it is a useful investigation and can be performed under aseptic conditions.

Norman J, Greer I, eds. Preterm labour: managing risk in clinical practice. Cambridge: Cambridge University Press; 2005.

RCOG Green-top Guideline 44. Preterm prelabour rupture of membranes; November 2006.

42. A. The baby's nappies should be changed on the floor

The risk of having a seizure in the first 24 hours post-delivery is 1–2%, so women should not be left unattended during this time. A lack of sleep in the post-partum period lowers the seizure threshold, so additional support is vital. To reduce the risk to the baby in the event of a seizure, nappy changes should be performed on the floor and the baby should be bathed in very shallow water. Vitamin K 1 mg intramuscular should be given to the baby to prevent haemorrhage.

Nelson-Piercy C. Handbook of obstetric medicine, 5th ed. New York: Informa Healthcare; 2015.

43. C. 40%

The risk of vertical transmission of CMV is 40% in the first and second trimester. Transmission occurs in about 80% of cases in the third trimester.

To M, Kidd M, Maxwell D. Prenatal diagnosis and management of fetal infections. TOG 2009;11:108–16.

44. C. Low birthweight

Knife cone biopsy increases the risk of preterm delivery, low birthweight, and CS.

Ellis P, Mould T. Fertility-saving treatment in gynaecological oncology. TOG 2009;11:239–44.

45. A. Allergic dermatitis

Allergic dermatitis is generally diagnosed from the history—a sudden and severe reaction is seen to an allergen such as nail polish, latex, or lanolin. Irritant dermatitis is triggered by an external agent such as a new detergent. Lichen simplex chronicus is identified by lichenification with exaggerated skin markings and excoriation. Herpes infection is usually unilateral.

Kingston A. The postmenopausal vulva. TOG 2009;11:253–9.

46. A. Intervals between menstruation of more than three months may be associated with endometrial hyperplasia

There is an increased risk of miscarriage both in PCOS and endometriosis patients compared to the general population. Oligo- or amenorrhoea in women with PCOS may predispose to endometrial hyperplasia and later carcinoma. In women with PCOS, intervals between menstruation of more than three months may be associated with endometrial hyperplasia. It is good practice to recommend treatment with progestogens to induce a withdrawal bleed at least every 3–4 months. Women who are oligomenorrhoeic and do not have normal withdrawal bleeds should be investigated by ultrasound scan, endometrial sampling, and hysteroscopy—whichever is or are appropriate according to the situation. There does not appear to be an association with breast or ovarian cancer, and no additional surveillance is required in this regard.

RCOG Green-top Guideline 33. Long-term consequences of polycystic ovary syndrome; 2014.

47. E. There is a higher risk of thromboembolism with GTN

Women with GTN will require single-agent chemotherapy if their FIGO 2000 score is 6 or less. The cure rate for women with a score of 6 or less is almost 100%, whilst the cure rate for women with a score greater than 7 is 95%. The age at menopause for women who receive single-agent chemotherapy is advanced by one year and by three years if they receive multiagent chemotherapy. Intrauterine devices should not be used until HCG levels are normal. This will reduce the risk of uterine perforation.

RCOG Green-top Guideline 38. Gestational trophoblastic disease; 2010.

48. A. *E. coli* urinary tract infection

Approximately 40% of spontaneous premature births are due to intrauterine infection. Asymptomatic bacteriuria, most commonly due to *Escherichia coli*, is often the cause. Other infective agents associated with preterm labour include gonococcal cervicitis, *Trichomonas vaginalis*, *Ureaplasma urealyticum*, *Mycoplasma hominis*, *Gardnerella vaginalis*, and bacteroides.

NICE Clinical Guideline 62. Antenatal care: routine care for the healthy pregnant woman; 2008 (updated in 2019).

NICE: Antenatal care NG201:2021

49. A. Lupus anticoagulant screening should be considered

A significant proportion of cases of recurrent miscarriage remain unexplained despite detailed investigation. These women can be reassured that the prognosis for a successful future pregnancy with supportive care alone is 75%. However, the prognosis worsens with increasing maternal age and number of previous miscarriages. Relevant investigations should be considered after two miscarriages especially among woman >35.

There is insufficient evidence to evaluate the effect of HCG supplementation in the treatment of recurrent miscarriage. A multicentre, placebo-controlled trial of HCG supplementation in early pregnancy failed to show any benefit for pregnancy outcome. There is now evidence to recommend progesterone supplementation in women with recurrent miscarriages for those who are Lupus anticoagulant negative. Progesterone supplementation should also be considered for women who presents with threatened miscarriage and have a viable pregnancy at ultrasound scan. Women with a history of second-trimester miscarriage and suspected cervical weakness who have not undergone a cerclage based on their history may be offered serial cervical sonographic surveillance. The live birth rate in women with unexplained recurrent miscarriage who conceive naturally is 20–30% higher than the live birth rate achieved after pre-implantation genetic screening or *in vitro* fertilization.

RCOG. New draft guideline outlines best practice for treating recurrent miscarriage; 2022.

Updated NICE guidance on miscarriage using progesterone to help prevent pregnancy loss (midirs. org); 2021.

50. D. Polyglycolic acid

Polyglycolic acid, or Dexon, is an absorbable braided synthetic polymer of glycolic acid. It is absorbed completely in 90–120 days. Polyglactin (Vicryl) is a synthetic multifilament heteropolymer which is fully degraded by hydrolysis within 90 days. Polypropylene (Prolene) is a synthetic monofilament non-absorbable suture.

Kudur M, et al. Sutures and suturing techniques in skin closure. *Indian J Dermatol Venereol Leprol* 2009;75:425–34.

Extended Matching Questions

Answers for Questions 1–5

1. D; 2. G; 3. I; 4. D; 5. L

1. This position cannot be delivered vaginally and therefore requires an emergency CS. She is 9 cm dilated and therefore requires delivery urgently but it would be safe for this to be within 60 minutes of the decision. Mento-anterior face presentations can deliver vaginally, delivering by the mechanism of extension rather than flexion. Mento-posterior cannot deliver vaginally as the head is already fully extended. Forceps can be applied to a mento-anterior face presentation by an experienced clinician.

2. All patients can have one hour for descent of the head after full dilatation is reached. This approach is more commonly practised in women with epidurals. Parous women should be encouraged to push for one hour before reassessment, whilst primigravidae should be encouraged to push for up to two hours before reassessment. If progress is being made then women can continue to push for one further hour with regular assessments at 15-minute intervals. This means that the second stage can be up to four hours long in a primigravida and three hours in a parous woman.

3. Exhaustion is an indication for assisted vaginal delivery. Ideally this woman would be encouraged to continue pushing for another 30 minutes before reassessment, but if she is unable to push effectively then assistance is required. She is fully dilated with a DOA position. She has sufficient analgesia (epidural). The choice is vacuum extraction or forceps delivery. Vacuum extraction has the advantage of causing less maternal tissue trauma and less maternal pain. However, it does require good maternal effort and is therefore not suitable in this circumstance.

4. Only one of the four features of a CTG is abnormal and therefore, the CTG should be classified as suspicious. This alongside the presence of meconium indicates that intervention is required. This would normally involve a foetal blood sample to determine management. However, in this scenario the woman is only at 32 weeks' gestation. FBS, FSE, vacuum extraction, and rotational forceps are contraindicated below 34 weeks, and therefore this patient should be delivered by CS.

5. There is no evidence here to indicate that this is a high-risk pregnancy. It would not be standard practice to offer a CTG in this situation, unless requested by the parents. The CTG is normal with all four features being reassuring, and therefore the CTG should be stopped. All of the other answers in this stem are interventions and none are appropriate. In practice, this woman would of course be reassured and offered appropriate pain relief with plans for reassessment.

NICE Clinical Guideline 132. Caesarean section; 2011.

NICE Clinical Guideline 55. Intra-partum care; 2007.

RCOG Green-top Guideline 26. Operative vaginal delivery; 2011.

Answers for Questions 6–10

6. N; 7. M; 8. L; 9. D; 10. B

6. Women with symptoms in early pregnancy suggestive of ectopic pregnancy or miscarriage should ideally attend a specialist early pregnancy unit. The introduction of such clinics with specialist trained nursing or midwifery staff and a dedicated ultrasound scanning facility have been proven to be highly cost-effective. Moreover, they are highly satisfactory in terms

of patient perception and they reduce the number of hospital admissions. Following the appropriate history and appropriate examination, all women should be offered chlamydia screening, have a serum HCG test, and have an ultrasound scan if the HCG is above the discriminatory zone. Transvaginal scanning is more accurate in early pregnancy, if tolerated by the patient.

7. This is a pregnancy of unknown location (PUL). Management options include medical or surgical management upon diagnosing the location of the pregnancy. If no mass can be seen on TVUSS, then it may not be possible to confidently identify an ectopic pregnancy during surgery. Surgery would expose the patient to the potential risks of surgery without providing proven treatment; rarely, surgery would result in the excision of a healthy tube. Methotrexate with monitoring of HCG response may be considered after USS confirmation of the location of the pregnancy by a senior clinician, especially as the patient has had previous abdominal surgery.

8. A repeat HCG is needed as the initial HCG is below the discriminatory zone. The trend in the HCG measurements is important: a doubling of HCG would suggest a normal pregnancy, a falling HCG may suggest a miscarriage, and a static HCG may indicate an ectopic pregnancy. There are of course exceptions to all of these rules! Read the question and all of the answers carefully before selecting your answer as there are often multiple similar answers.

9. The scenario suggests a ruptured ectopic pregnancy with an unstable patient. It is important to demonstrate that you acknowledge that this woman requires urgent surgery to stop the bleeding. Guidelines suggest that management in an acute situation would likely be by laparotomy rather than laparoscopically.

10. The patient is clinically stable and has a diagnosis of ectopic pregnancy. As she wishes to avoid surgery, medical management with methotrexate would be the obvious answer. However, she does not fulfil the criteria for methotrexate as she has a live ectopic; therefore, surgery is her only option. As she is stable, a laparoscopic approach would be suitable.

NICE Guideline NG126. Ectopic pregnancy and miscarriage: diagnosis and initial management. 17 April 2019; last updated: 24 November 2021.

RCOG Green-top Guideline 21. Management of tubal pregnancy, 2004.

Answers for Questions 11–15

11. J; 12.B; 13. M; 14. H; 15. G

11. Extra mammary Paget's disease is usually seen in white postmenopausal women and can be associated with an underlying adenocarcinoma. The rash is classically described as 'strawberries and cream' owing to the extensive erythema, often with lichenification and excoriation. Other extramammary sites include the eyelids, axilla, perianal region, mons pubis, and glans penis.

12. Vulval candidiasis presents with irritation and soreness of the vulva and anus, superficial dyspareunia, and occasionally vaginal discharge. The majority of infections are caused by *Candida albicans*. Risk factors include diabetes, obesity, and antibiotic use. On examination, there may be oedema and fissuring with satellite lesions extending out from the labia majora to the inner thighs or mons pubis in chronic cases. The discharge may be described as 'curdy' or 'cottage-cheese-like'. Prolonged topical or oral antifungal therapy may be necessary to clear infections.

13. The majority of cases of VIN are of the 'usual type'. There are three subgroups: warty, basaloid, and mixed. It is most commonly seen between the ages of 35 and 55 years. It can

present with pruritus, dyspareunia, or a visible lesion, although up to 50% are asymptomatic. It is associated with HPV infection and premalignant disease of the genital and anal area. Other risk factors include smoking and chronic immunosuppression. Usual-type VIN is classically multicentric and multifocal; its colour and appearance can vary widely.

14. Anogenital lichen sclerosus is most commonly seen in postmenopausal women but can occur at any age including prior to puberty. The main symptom is severe pruritus, which may be worse at night. Trauma from scratching may result in bleeding and pain including dyspareunia. Aetiology is thought to be autoimmune and not linked to hormones. On examination, the whole vulval perianal area may be affected with a classic distribution of 'figure-of-eight'. The skin is often atrophic and may show ecchymoses, adhesions, and a smooth, shiny parchment-like or cigarette-paper-like appearance. Chronic disease results in distortion of anatomy, which may include fusion and reabsorption of the labia minora and burying of the clitoris, and in severe cases may precipitate difficulty with micturition, retention, or both.

15. Lichen planus (LP) is difficult to differentiate from lichen sclerosus. In LP the vaginal introitus is usually involved. Adhesions and erosions may occur and be unresponsive to surgical division. Oral and gingival involvement is possible.

British Association for Sexual Health and HIV national guideline for the management of vulvovaginal candidiasis (2019); 2020 (sagepub.com).

Edwards SK, Bates CM, Lewis F, Sethi G, Grover D. 2014 UK national guideline on the management of vulval conditions. *Int J STD AIDS* 2015;26(9):611–24.

RCOG Green-top Guideline 58. The management of vulval skin disorders; 2011.

Rogers CA, Beardall AJ. Recurrent vulvovaginal candidiasis. *Int J STD AIDS* 1999;10:435–41.

Answers for Questions 16–20

16. M; 17. I; 18. P; 19. N; 20. J

16. Good history-taking and bladder diaries are sufficiently reliable to categorize urinary incontinence and plan initial non-invasive treatment decisions. A trial of supervised pelvic floor exercise for at least three months duration and bladder training for a minimum of six weeks should be offered as the first-line of treatment to women with stress or mixed incontinence. The POPPY trial also showed that physiotherapy is useful in the management of prolapse.

17. Many different treatments have been proposed but none have been proven to be completely effective. If therapy with non-steroidal anti-inflammatory agents and long-term antibiotics has failed, therapy with bladder-coating agents such as intravesical hyaluronic acid (Cystistat) has been shown to be beneficial.

18. Carrying out urodynamic investigations before initial treatment for stress incontinence has not been shown to improve outcome. However, it is of value if the initial surgical treatment has failed.

19. This woman has tried conservative measures for her presumed stress incontinence and seeks definitive treatment. She has stress incontinence complicated by urgency, so standard cystometry would be the investigation of choice prior to surgery.

20. Although the presentation could be consistent with detrusor overactivity, these symptoms could also indicate an ovarian mass. An ultrasound examination of abdomen and pelvis is indicated before further investigation of her urinary symptoms.

NICE Clinical Guideline 171. Urinary incontinence in women: management; 11 September 2013; last updated: 5 November 2015.

Answers for Questions 21–25

21. I; 22. F; 23. C; 24. A; 25. E

21. Painless cervical dilatation and miscarriage during the second trimester suggests cervical incompetence and preterm pre-rupture of membranes. This patient should be counselled that she will have an ultrasound cervical assessment during second trimester, with a prophylactic first-trimester cervical cerclage.

22. Tubal patency assessment for a parous infertile woman with no history of pelvic infection, pelvic inflammatory disease, or pelvic endometriosis should be by hysterosalpingogram as the first-line investigation. Given the history, laparoscopy is indicated in this case.

23. Women with primary infertility with complex histories, especially those with irregular bleeding and deep dyspareunia, are at higher risk of pelvic endometriosis. Such patients should be investigated by diagnostic laparoscopy to assess any concomitant comorbidity which needs to be treated. Furthermore, she will benefit from a diagnostic hysteroscopy if periods have been irregular in order to rule out a submucous fibroid or multiple polypi. Remember that endometriosis and uterine fibroids are oestrogen-dependent conditions.

24. This patient's main problem is anovulation and initially she should be treated with an anti-oestrogen such as clomiphene to ensure that her cycles become ovulatory. Once she has demonstrable ovulatory cycles, then tubal patency can be checked.

25. This patient's main problem relates to the male factor and most likely she will be offered IUI with donor semen. Hysterosalpingogram should be offered to confirm tubal patency before starting intrauterine insemination treatment.

NICE Clinical Guideline 156. Fertility problems: assessment and treatment; 20 February 2013; last updated 6 September 2017.

Answers for Questions 26–30

26. K; 27. A; 28. M; 29. C; 30. K

26. As this patient had normal investigations, including thrombophilia screening, she should be reassured and advised to take folic acid.

27. This patient should be treated with low-molecular-weight heparin. There is evidence to suggest that the pregnancy outcome is better when patients are offered low-molecular-weight heparin and low-dose aspirin throughout pregnancy compared to either low-dose aspirin alone or low molecular weight heparin alone.

28. Obesity is an independent risk factor for recurrent pregnancy loss. As this woman has a normal thrombophilia screen, she should be encouraged to lose weight. There is no convincing evidence that metformin will improve conception rate.

29. Surgical termination during the second trimester increases the risk of cervical damage and thus increases the risk of preterm pre-rupture of membranes. Therefore such patients should be offered cervical length assessment by ultrasound scan during the first trimester and be followed-up by serial scan assessment during the second trimester.

30. All investigations are normal. Arcuate uterus does not increase the risk of miscarriage; therefore uterine reconstructive surgery has a very limited role. This patient should therefore be reassured.

Chan Y, et al. Reproductive uterine outcomes in women with congenital uterine anomalies: A systemic review. *Ultrasound Obstet Gynecol* 2011;38:371–82.

RCOG Green-top Guideline 17. Recurrent miscarriage: investigations and treatment of couples; 2011.

Answers for Questions 31–35

31. A; 32. E; 33. F; 34. D; 35. H

31. An unstable lie in a multiparous woman is a cause for concern because of the risk of malpresentation or cord prolapse when the membranes rupture. Admission until delivery is indicated, but may not be accepted by a woman with responsibilities for four existing offspring. It may be possible to perform a stabilizing ARM nearer to full term.

32. In a low-risk multiparous woman, an ECV is indicated.

33. ECV is not appropriate due to the previous scars on her uterus. As this will be her third CS and sixth child, long-term contraception should be discussed.

34. This woman can be reassured that the presentation is almost certain to be cephalic now and a rapid presentation scan in the clinic will demonstrate this to her. The sensitive obstetrician might wish to explore the background to her excessive anxiety and may also wish to probe the reasons why the community midwife was unable to give her the necessary reassurance and support. The woman should be discharged back to midwife-led care. If the presentation is found to be breech after 34 weeks, she may be referred back to the antenatal clinic.

35. Delivery is imminent, so vaginal breech delivery is an option. However, as this is a preterm labour, steroids should be considered. As membranes have ruptured and she is >4 cm dilated, tocolysis is not appropriate.

RCOG Green-top Guideline 20a. External cephalic version and reducing the incidence of breech presentation; 2006.

RCOG Green-top Guideline 20b. Management of breech presentation; 2006, last reviewed 2017.

Answers for Questions 36–40

36. J; 37. G; 38. C; 39. H; 40. I

36. Specificity is the ability of a test to identify the absence of a disease when the disease really is not present; that is, the proportion negative of those who do not have the disease.

37. The positive predictive value (PPV) is the proportion of subjects with positive test results who actually have the disease. Note that there is no consensus on the proportion of false-positive or false-negative rates, so it should be made clear exactly what is being calculated.

38. The false-positive rate is the proportion of patients who screen positive but do not actually have the disease. For example, a mammogram may suggest a positive signal for a cancer lesion but the biopsy is negative.

39. The screen-positive rate is the proportion of individuals in a given population reported to be positive on screening. It can be age-specific (e.g. X% of women under the age of 25 were screen positive for chlamydia), or ethnic-group-specific (e.g. X% of women under the age of 40 in the Asian population had an abnormal GTT).

40. Sensitivity is the ability of a test to identify a disease when it is really present; that is, the proportion of patients having the disease who test positive.

Gardner M, Altman D. *Statistics with confidence.* London: BMJ Press; 2013

Answers for Questions 41–45

41. A; 42. F; 43. C; 44. B; 45. J

41. A surgical option is suggested in view of her age and good state of health. Although both abdominal sacropexy and sacrospinous vault fixation would be reasonable options, the former may be the optimum procedure because recurrence risks are lower and dyspareunia is less likely than with the vaginal procedure.

42. A pessary is unlikely to be retained, due to the posterior prolapse. A repeat standard posterior repair is unlikely to be successful in view of the rapid recurrence following the first procedure. A mesh-augmented posterior repair would have been a choice in the past. Posterior repair with sacrospinous fixation is an alternative choice.

43. A pessary will not provide the desired definitive treatment. Although a standard anterior vaginal wall repair is an option, the recurrence risks can be very high, and future surgery may prove difficult if her family responsibilities intensify. Use of a mesh to augment the anterior repair might limit the risk of recurrence but carries a significant risk that her sexual life will be disrupted. A paravaginal repair carries a higher success rate than a standard anterior repair and may have fewer long-term side effects than a mesh procedure.

44. Colpocleisis is a good option here, provided sexual function does not need to be retained. Success rates are high.

45. Traditional anterior repair is the optimal procedure for this woman.

NICE Clinical Guideline 171. The management of urinary incontinence in women; 2013.

Answers for Questions 46–50

46. F; 47. G; 48. H; 49. D; 50. I

46. A deputy is appointed by the court to make decisions for someone who lacks mental capacity—someone who can't make a decision for themselves at the time it needs to be made. They may still be able to make decisions at other times. People may lack mental capacity due to dementia or because they have had a serious brain injury or illness.

    There are two types of deputy, depending on whether they make decisions about (a) property and financial affairs (e.g. paying bills, organizing a pension) or (b) personal welfare (e.g. care and medical treatment).

47. Lasting power of attorney means you can make, or help to make, decisions about someone's property and money if they appointed you to this position. A lasting (or enduring) power of attorney can help manage a variety of concerns, including money and bills, bank and building society accounts, property and investments, and pensions and benefits (https://www.gov.uk/enduring-power-attorney-duties).

48. The Office of the Public Guardian (OPG) protects people in England and Wales who may not have the mental capacity to make certain decisions for themselves, such as about their health finances. The OPG publishes annual reports.

49. The Court of Protection makes decisions on applications which involve people who lack mental capacity. The Mental Health Act applies to England and Wales and provides a framework to empower and protect people who may lack capacity to make certain decisions for themselves. The court of protection can make decisions in relation to serious medical treatment cases which relate to providing, withholding, or withdrawing treatment from a person who lacks capacity (https://www.gov.uk/court-of-protection).

50. The procurator fiscal in Scotland, or procurator coroner in England and Wales, is an independent judicial office holder, usually with a legal background, appointed by the local council. The coroner investigates deaths that appear violent or unnatural, and when the cause of death is unknown. By law, all maternal and neonatal deaths must be reported to this office.

General Medical Council. Management for doctors. Available at: https://www.gmc.org.uk

RCOG: StratOG. Clinical Governance e-tutorial. The obstetrician and gynaecologist as a professional. Available at: https:// www.rcog.org.uk.

Single Best Answers

1. **You are asked to review the summative assessments within obstetrics and gynaecology by your educational supervisor. Which ONE of the following is an example of a summative assessment?**

   A. Case-based discussion
   B. Induction interview
   C. Mini-clinical evaluation exercise
   D. Recruitment interview
   E. Team observation 1 form (form TO1)

2. **A 60-year-old woman presents with a change in bowel habit and abdominal swelling. An ultrasound scan suggests bilateral complex ovarian cysts and her RMI is 400. What is her risk of ovarian cancer?**

   A. 20%
   B. 35%
   C. 50%
   D. 65%
   E. 75%

3. **A 24-year-old insulin-dependent diabetic woman in her first pregnancy asks you what the impact of persistent high blood glucose is on her baby at birth. Which ONE of the following is the correct impact?**

   A. Anaemia
   B. Hypercalcaemia
   C. Hyperglycaemia
   D. Hypobilirubinaemia
   E. Respiratory distress syndrome

4. **A 19-year-old woman presents with a fever four days after a normal vaginal delivery. She is diagnosed with tuberculosis. How would you treat the baby?**
    A. Administer Bacille–Calmette–Guerin vaccination
    B. Administer isoniazid
    C. Administer isoniazid and vitamin B6
    D. No treatment is needed for the baby, but avoid breastfeeding
    E. No treatment is needed for the baby, but treat the mother

5. **You are asked to review a 27-year-old Jehovah's Witness in her first pregnancy at 24 weeks gestation. Which ONE of the following recommendations is she most likely to accept in the event of a massive obstetric haemorrhage?**
    A. Autologous blood transfusion
    B. Plasma infusion
    C. Platelet transfusion
    D. Red cell transfusion
    E. Whole blood transfusion

6. **You review a 23-year-old primiparous woman at 26 weeks gestation with known cytomegalovirus (CMV) infection. What is the laboratory finding in a foetus with congenital CMV infection?**
    A. Haemolytic anaemia
    B. High urea
    C. Hypoalbuminaemia
    D. Microcephaly
    E. Neutropenia

7. **A GP refers a 47-year-old woman with a suspicion of VIN. What is the most common symptom associated with VIN?**
    A. Bleeding
    B. Pain
    C. Pruritus
    D. Ulceration
    E. White, thick skin plaques

8. **A 30-year-old nulliparous woman is referred to you complaining of cyclical pelvic pain and abdominal swelling. A pelvic ultrasound suggests a diagnosis of adenomyosis. What is your first-line management?**
    A. Hysterectomy
    B. The levonorgestrel-releasing intrauterine system
    C. Norethisterone
    D. Tranexamic acid
    E. Uterine ablation

9. **A 27-year-old woman presents at 29 + 4 weeks gestation with vaginal spotting. An ultrasound report confirms a high anterior placenta and when you review her there is no bleeding. She reports good foetal movements. What is your management plan?**

   A. Admit for observation
   B. Admit until 24 hours have passed since the last episode of spotting
   C. Observe for 4–6 hours and if clinically well, discharge home
   D. Reassure and discharge home
   E. Review in the maternal assessment unit within 24 hours

10. **You are clearing your in-tray and come across several patient results of investigations requested by your team. On reviewing a semen analysis result, which ONE of the following parameters is normal?**

    A. Normal forms 4%
    B. Semen volume 1 ml
    C. Sperm concentration 15×10^5/ml
    D. Total motility 40%
    E. Total number of sperm 20×10^6/ml

11. **You counsel a 19-year-old woman who has been diagnosed with PCOS on the benefits of the combined oral contraceptive pill (COCP). Which ONE of the following is a non-contraceptive benefit of the COCP?**

    A. It protects against gallstones
    B. Reduction in intermenstrual bleeding
    C. Reduction in the risk of cervical cancer
    D. Reduction in the risk of colorectal cancer
    E. Reduction in the size of ovarian endometriomas

12. **A 26-year-old primiparous woman presents with her second episode of reduced foetal movements at 30 weeks gestation. What is your first line of management?**

    A. Assess the amniotic fluid index
    B. Ask the patient to lie on their left side for 20 minutes
    C. Perform a CTG
    D. Request an umbilical artery Doppler velocity
    E. Request biophysical profiling

13. **You are reviewing the histology results for patients who have presented to the rapid access clinic. Which ONE of the following is correct?**

    A. Atypical hyperplasia can be managed conservatively
    B. Complex hyperplasia should be monitored every six months
    C. Cystic hyperplasia can be treated by uterine curettage
    D. Progestogens should be avoided in adenomatous hyperplasia
    E. An ultrasound should be performed to exclude endogenous oestrogen in women with atypical hyperplasia

14. **Which ONE of the following statements is true of perinatal mortality?**

    A. The 2020 MBRRACE-UK Perinatal Mortality Surveillance Report noted a 19% increase in twin stillbirth rate
    B. Birth trauma represents the third most common cause of neonatal deaths in the UK in 2008
    C. In the UK, intrapartum stillbirths are responsible for most of the stillbirths
    D. In the UK, perinatal death is defined as the death of a foetus or a newborn in the perinatal period that commences at 22 completed weeks gestation and ends before seven completed days after birth
    E. The Wigglesworth and Aberdeen obstetric classifications of stillbirths identify over 80% of causes of stillbirth

15. **A 32-year-old woman comes to see you following her second pregnancy, which resulted following contraceptive failure. All of the following contraceptive methods primarily work by inhibiting ovulation, except for**

    A. The combined hormonal contraceptive pill (CHC)
    B. The combined vaginal ring (CVR)
    C. Depot medroxyprogesterone acetate (DMPA)
    D. The levonorgesterel-containing intrauterine system (IUS)
    E. The subdermal contraceptive implant

16. **A 37-year-old woman presents at 38 weeks gestation with reduced foetal movements. This is her fourth pregnancy. Ultrasound confirms an intrauterine foetal death. Which ONE investigation is the single most important test when investigating late intrauterine foetal death?**

    A. Foetal skin biopsy
    B. Kleihauer test
    C. Maternal coagulation profile and plasma fibrinogen
    D. MRI
    E. Post-mortem examination of the cord, membranes, and placenta

17. **You are asked to review a 26-year-old woman in the antenatal clinic with regard to the impact of her medical history on the duration of the second stage of labour. Which ONE of the following medical conditions requires a shorter second stage?**

    A. Asthma
    B. Knee arthritis
    C. Pre-eclampsia requiring antihypertensive therapy
    D. The presence of ocular chorioretinitis
    E. Spinal cord injury

18. **A 54-year-old woman presents following one episode of postmenopausal bleeding. You note she is on tamoxifen. What type of drug is tamoxifen?**
    A. ACE inhibitor
    B. Dopamine antagonist
    C. Progesterone antagonist
    D. Selective oestrogen receptor modulator
    E. Testosterone inhibitor

19. **A 33-year-old woman is referred urgently following a diagnosis of breast cancer. She is 14 weeks gestation in her second pregnancy. Which ONE of the following is true regarding breast cancer in pregnancy?**
    A. Breast cancer affects 1 in 300 pregnant women
    B. Breastfeeding should be avoided
    C. Pre-eclampsia is a protective factor
    D. Pregnancy should be deferred for one year after diagnosis
    E. Tamoxifen can be given in the second and third trimesters

20. **You review a 29-year-old HIV-positive woman who is 27 weeks pregnant. She is on zidovudine. What type of drug is this?**
    A. Cytokine
    B. Non-nucleoside reverse transcriptase inhibitor
    C. Nucleoside reverse transcriptase inhibitor
    D. Nucleoside reverse transcriptase potentiator
    E. Protease inhibitor

21. **A 27-year-old woman attended for her detailed foetal anomaly scan at 20 weeks. The scan was performed by an ultrasonographer, who notes the foetal femur length is below the 10th centile. What advice would you give her?**
    A. Advise foetal karyotyping
    B. Advise termination of pregnancy
    C. Arrange serial growth scans
    D. Reassure and treat as normal pregnancy
    E. Repeat scan in two weeks

22. **A 35-year-old nulliparous woman and her partner present in the clinic to discuss IVF. Which ONE of the following statements is true regarding the success of IVF?**
    A. Caffeine intake by women undergoing assisted conception does not reduce the live birth rate
    B. IVF is more successful in women who have had a previous pregnancy
    C. IVF is the method of choice for men with oligozoospermia
    D. Maternal BMI has no effect on the success of IVF
    E. Smoking by the male partner is not associated with a reduced live birth rate in IVF treatment

23. **Which ONE of the following is true regarding preterm prelabour rupture of membranes:**

    A. Chorioamnionitis commonly presents with symptoms of pyrexia, uterine tenderness, and foul-smelling liquor
    B. Full blood count and C-reactive protein tests have high sensitivity for the detection of chorioamnionitis
    C. Once the diagnosis has been established, weekly high vaginal swabs should be performed to detect chorioamnionitis early
    D. Tests such as rapid immunoassay AmniSure® have a specificity of 100% and sensitivity of 99%
    E. Ultrasound examination is the most accurate investigation to confirm the diagnosis of preterm prelabour rupture of membranes (PPROM)

24. **A 39-year-old woman has been referred for a cervical smear. She underwent a cervical biopsy at the age of 32, but all smears have been normal since then. Which ONE of the following statements is correct regarding cervical screening?**

    A. Cervical smears can be discontinued at 60 years
    B. Colposcopically directed punch biopsy should be performed if the transformational zone appears atypical
    C. If routine cervical screening is due and if a woman falls pregnant cervical smear should be performed
    D. If the recent cervical smear has shown abnormality and if the woman is now pregnant referral to colposcopy after delivery is recommended
    E. Screening interval does not depend on the age group

25. **A 25-year-old woman with hyperthyroidism presents in her first pregnancy. Which ONE of the following is true regarding treatment?**

    A. Beta blockers can cause tremor
    B. It is safe to breastfeed while on propylthiouracil (PTU)
    C. PTU does not cross the placenta whereas carbimazole does
    D. PTU is associated with foetal aplasia cutis
    E. Radioactive iodine is safe in breastfeeding

26. **A 36-year-old multiparous woman presents with urinary incontinence on coughing and sneezing. She has a background history of ulcerative colitis and tried physiotherapy but this has not helped. Which ONE of the following is licensed for use to manage stress urinary incontinence?**

    A. Botulinum toxin A
    B. Darifenacin
    C. Duloxetine
    D. Oxybutynin
    E. Sertraline

27. **In which ONE of the following cases would a cervical cerclage be suitable?**

    A. A 24-year-old woman with a DCDA twin pregnancy; ultrasound indicates a cervical length of 2 cm at 16 weeks
    B. A 27-year-old woman with a history of two preterm deliveries
    C. A 30-year-old woman with a history of painless miscarriage at 23 weeks
    D. A 36-year-old woman who has an incidental finding of a cervical length of 25 mm at anomaly ultrasound
    E. A 38-year-old woman in her first pregnancy with PPROM

28. **A 27-year-old woman is suspected to have a partial molar pregnancy. Which ONE of the following management options is correct?**

    A. Perform surgical evacuation, with oxytocin administered prior to completing the evacuation
    B. MRI should be performed to exclude metastases
    C. An ultrasound scan is required to make a definitive diagnosis
    D. Upon surgical evacuation, partial moles are found to have foetal tissue or foetal red blood cells present
    E. Women with gestational trophoblastic neoplasia will require radiotherapy

29. **A 24-year-old primigravida woman is diagnosed to have a twin pregnancy. Which ONE of the following is correct?**

    A. Laser ablation is the preferred treatment for twin-to-twin transfusion syndrome (TTTS) at 28 weeks
    B. The risk of twin stillbirth is over twice that of singletons
    C. The risk of foetal loss is higher in MCMA pregnancies
    D. The 'twin peak' sign on ultrasound is diagnostic of DCDA twins
    E. TTTS complicates 15% of DCDA pregnancies

30. **A 28-year-old woman at 26 weeks gestation is referred to see you in the antenatal clinic with a history of genital herpes. Which ONE of the following is correct?**

    A. Foetal scalp electrodes and foetal blood sampling in labour are to be avoided in a woman with recurrent genital herpes
    B. Local central nervous system disease (encephalitis alone), one of the subgroups of neonatal herpes, often present late and is associated with a mortality rate of 6% and neurological morbidity of 70% if treated
    C. The most common route of transmission of the virus is by contact with maternal secretions
    D. Recurrent episodes of genital herpes during the antenatal period warrant elective delivery by caesarean section
    E. Recurrent episodes of genital herpes are associated with a 3% risk of neonatal herpes, even if lesions are present at the time of delivery

31. **A 57-year-old multiparous woman presents after an episode of heavy vaginal bleeding. Ultrasound shows a regular endometrium, with a thickness of 5 mm. However, a 9 cm irregular ovarian mass is seen in the left adnexal area. What is the most likely tumour type?**
    A. Clear cell tumour
    B. Granulosa cell tumour
    C. Mucinous cell tumour
    D. Sertoli-Leydig tumour
    E. Transitional cell carcinoma

32. **You are called urgently by your SHO to review a 24-year-old woman with critical ovarian hyperstimulation syndrome (OHSS). Which ONE of the following features suggests critical OHSS?**
    A. Haematocrit greater than 45%
    B. Hyponatraemia
    C. Mild oliguria
    D. Ovarian size 8–12 cm
    E. White cell count greater than 17,000/ml

33. **A 42-year-old woman and her partner present to the infertility clinic following a miscarriage at eight weeks gestation. This is her second first-trimester miscarriage; they have a five-year-old son. Which ONE of the following is true regarding recurrent miscarriage?**
    A. The age-related risk of miscarriage in women more than 45 years is over 90%
    B. Antiphospholipid antibodies are present in 1% of women who experience recurrent miscarriage
    C. In women with unexplained recurrent miscarriage, preimplantation genetic screening followed by in-vitro fertilization increases live birth rates
    D. It affects 5% of couples
    E. Paternal age is not a risk factor for miscarriage

34. **You review a 25-year-old woman who is 32 weeks pregnant. She has been diagnosed to have human parvovirus B19 infection. Which ONE of the following is the clinical manifestation seen in the foetus?**
    A. Chorioretinitis
    B. Intrauterine growth restriction
    C. Microcephaly
    D. Non-immune hydrops
    E. Oligohydramnios

35. A 61-year-old woman presents with urge incontinence symptoms after surgical treatment for stress incontinence. Following colposuspension, the rate of de novo detrusor overactivity is

A. 5%

B. 15%

C. 30%

D. 40%

E. 60%

36. A 29-year-old woman presents with a two-year history of worsening vulvodynia. What treatment would you advocate first line?

A. Amitryptyline

B. Clobetasol propionate

C. Cognitive behaviour therapy

D. Flucloxacillin

E. Topical steroids

37. You review the booking blood test results of a 34-year-old multiparous woman. She has a positive HIV test. What immediate advice will you give her?

A. She should be offered HIV testing of older children if their HIV status is unknown

B. She should not have invasive testing, such as amniocentesis

C. She should take aspirin throughout the pregnancy

D. She will need antiretroviral medication throughout her pregnancy

E. She will need delivery by caesarean section

38. A 33-year-old multiparous woman presents at 38 weeks gestation with breech presentation. She would like a vaginal breech delivery. Which ONE of the following factors is unfavourable for vaginal breech birth?

A. Estimated foetal weight below tenth centile

B. Frank breech presentation

C. Poorly controlled gestational diabetes

D. The presence of 5 cm fundal fibroid

E. Previous history of PPH

39. Non-genital injuries have been reported in up to 80% of victims of sexual assault. Which ONE of the following statements correctly describes the characteristic features of the given injury?

A. Ecchymoses are pinpoint haemorrhages produced by rupture of small blood vessels (venules) by physical trauma

B. Erythema results from extravasation of blood into soft tissue as a result of blunt trauma

C. Lacerations are caused by a tangential force, which removes the superficial epithelial layers of the dermis

D. Slash wounds show an irregular contour, bruising to the edges, and tissue strands such as nerves and fibrous bands crossing in the depth of the wound

E. Stab wounds are injuries that are deeper than they are long and have sharp wound edges

40. **A 20-year-old woman presents with a unilateral 6 cm ovarian mass. Ultrasound scan notes hyperechoic areas with a mass suggestive of bone. She is admitted to the gynaecology ward with severe abdominal pain. On examination, she has guarding and rebound. Which ONE of the following is the likely nature of the ovarian mass?**

A. Dysgerminoma

B. Immature malignant teratoma

C. Mature cystic teratoma

D. Primary ovarian choriocarcinoma

E. Struma ovarii

41. **You discuss ulipristal acetate (UPA)-containing emergency contraception for a 24-year-old woman requesting emergency contraception. Which ONE of the following is correct?**

A. A double dose should be given if the woman is using liver enzyme-inducing medication

B. It can be administered beyond 120 hours

C. It is considered first line for women taking antacids or H_2 receptor antagonists

D. It can be used more than once in the same menstrual cycle

E. The primary mechanism of action is prevention of implantation

42. **You review a 57-year-old woman with an 8 cm complex ovarian mass and ascites. You are about to place her on the operating list when your consultant asks you for her RMI. Which ONE of the following features of the ultrasound scan contributes to the RMI?**

A. Evidence of fluid levels within the cyst

B. Multilocular cyst

C. Poor colour Doppler flow

D. Thickened endometrium

E. Unilateral lesions

43. **In the treatment of endometriosis, which ONE of the following is true:**

A. Cases of severe endometriosis should be managed surgically only

B. Endometriosis is a progressive condition in more than 80% of cases

C. Laparoscopic incision of endometriomas with drainage and irrigation is associated with low morbidity but more pain recurrence than excision

D. Medical treatment of laparoscopically diagnosed endometriosis improves the likelihood of conception

E. Surgical excision of mild to moderate endometriosis has poorer outcomes in comparison to other treatment modalities

44. **A 56-year-old woman undergoes urodynamic assessment. During the test, there is no change to detrusor activity; however, she experiences urinary leaking on coughing. The diagnosis is therefore most likely to be:**
    A. Medication-related
    B. Mixed urinary incontinence
    C. Stress urinary incontinence
    D. Urge urinary incontinence
    E. Urinary tract infection

45. **A 23-year-old woman presents with a headache and history of feeling unwell over the last 36 hours. You note her temperature is 38.5 °C. Blood investigations reveal a platelet count of 70×10⁹/L and abnormal renal function. Which ONE of the following is the diagnosis?**
    A. HELLP syndrome
    B. Immune thrombocytopenic purpura
    C. Lymphoma
    D. Thrombotic thrombocytopaenic purpura
    E. Viral infection

46. **A 34-year-old woman with a BMI of 34 presents for contraceptive advice. She has had treatment for a DVT. Concerning hormonal contraception and thromboembolic disease, which ONE of the following is true?**
    A. For women who are post-partum and not breastfeeding, combined hormonal contraception can be started immediately
    B. For women with current venous thromboembolism on anticoagulants, the progestogen-only pill is contraindicated
    C. Hormonal contraception can be started immediately after a first- or second-trimester termination of pregnancy
    D. Progestogen-only pills, implants, and the levonorgestrel-releasing intrauterine system have an increased risk of venous thromboembolism
    E. Women with factor V Leiden have up to a fivefold increase in the risk of VTE with combined oral contraceptive use

47. **A 27-year-old woman is referred to see you urgently with an abnormal-looking cervix and smear. Which ONE of the following is correct?**
    A. 1B tumours are not usually obvious on examination
    B. 1B2 tumours are at least 2 cm in size
    C. Bilateral salpingo-oophorectomy should be performed in all women with adenocarcinoma of the cervix
    D. HPV subtypes 16 and 18 are associated with the development of cervical cancer
    E. Smoking is the main risk factor for the development of cervical cancer

48. You are performing a preoperative gynaecology ward round. Regarding consent, which **ONE** of the following is true?

A. A complication which occurs less than 1 in 10,000 is rare

B. The need for repeat surgical evacuation after SMM is up to almost 20 in 1,000 women

C. Non-surgical methods are associated with a higher risk of infection compared to surgical evacuation of the uterus

D. Non-surgical methods are associated with up to a 25% possibility of eventually needing surgical evacuation

E. A serious risk of surgical evacuation of the uterus is localized pelvic infection

49. You are reviewing a 34-year-old multiparous woman who presents to antenatal clinic at 37 weeks gestation with breech presentation. External cephalic version has failed and she would like to finalize her birth plan for vaginal breech delivery. Which **ONE** of the following would you advise?

A. Delivery can occur in the midwifery-led unit

B. Early epidural analgesia should be advised

C. An episiotomy will be required in all cases

D. Induction of labour should not be considered

E. Labour augmentation with syntocinon should not be considered

50. A 60-year-old woman presents with constant runny vaginal discharge, smelling of urine. She underwent brachytherapy for cervical cancer four months ago and you suspect a vesico-vaginal fistula. A vesico-vaginal fistula can be most accurately visualized using:

A. CT

B. Micturating cystourethrography

C. MRI

D. Plain abdominal radiograph

E. Ultrasound

Extended Matching Questions

Options for Questions 1–5

The list of options describes appropriate risk frequencies associated with recurrent pregnancy loss. For each of the following clinical scenarios, choose the most appropriate risk frequency. Each option may be used once, more than once, or not at all.

    A. 11%
    B. 12%
    C. 13%
    D. 15%
    E. 25%
    F. 35%
    G. 40%
    H. 51%
    I. 60%
    J. 75%
    K. 80%
    L. 85%
    M. 93%

1. A 24-year-old woman presents to preconception clinic with a normal BMI. What is her risk of having a miscarriage?
2. A 35-year-old healthy woman attends an infertility clinic. What is her risk of miscarriage?
3. What is the lifetime risk of a further first-trimester pregnancy loss for a 30-year-old woman who has had three first-trimester miscarriages?
4. What is the age-related risk of miscarriage for a 43-year-old nulliparous woman?
5. What is the age-related risk of miscarriage for a 46-year-old nulliparous woman?

Options for Questions 6–9

For each of the following clinical scenarios, choose the most appropriate management. Each option may be used once, more than once, or not at all.

    A. Aspirin
    B. Codeine phosphate
    C. GnRH agonist
    D. GnRH antagonist
    E. Hartmann's solution
    F. HCG
    G. HCG and GnRH agonist
    H. Human albumin solution
    I. Hypertonic saline
    J. Insulin
    K. Metformin
    L. Morphine
    M. Normal saline

6. A 36-year-old woman with moderate OHSS complains of generalized abdominal discomfort, with no pain relief despite taking paracetamol.

7. A 35-year-old woman has been admitted to the acute gynaecology unit three days following an embryo transfer. Her haemoglobin is 130 and her haematocrit is 49%. Her sodium levels are 128. What fluid would be the most appropriate for her?

8. A 38-year-old woman with a BMI 35 and with PCOS is due to undergo IVF. What additional drug might be considered during her stimulation to reduce the risk of OHSS?

9. A 38-year-old, para 0 + 0, is coming for a second IVF cycle. She had severe OHSS during the first treatment cycle. What drug regimen should be used for down-regulation for her current treatment cycle?

Options for Questions 10–14

For each of the following clinical scenarios, choose the most appropriate response. Each option may be used once, more than once, or not at all.

A. Common perineal nerve
B. Femoral nerve
C. Genito-femoral nerve
D. Ileo-hypogastric nerve
E. Ileo-inguinal nerve
F. Lateral cutaneous nerve
G. Obturator nerve
H. Pudendal nerve
I. Sciatic nerve
J. Tibial nerve

10. A 40-year-old woman underwent a total abdominal hysterectomy and bilateral salpingo-oophorectomy for severe endometriosis. On day three following the operation, she complains of weakness of hip flexion. On examination the knee jerk reflex is absent and paraesthesia is present over the anterior and medial thigh.

11. A 60-year-old woman with a BMI of 40 had a total abdominal hysterectomy and bilateral salpingo-oophorectomy through a Pfannenstiel incision for a pelvic mass. She is now complaining of sharp burning pain radiating from the incision site to the labia and thigh.

12. A 38-year-old woman underwent extensive surgery for carcinoma cervix stage 1B with lymph node dissection. She is now complaining of paraesthesia over the labia majorum and femoral triangle.

13. A 70-year-old woman who has previously had a hysterectomy had a vaginal procedure to correct vault prolapse. She is now complaining of gluteal, vulval, and perineal pain while seated.

14. A 40-year-old woman underwent the insertion of a transobturator tape. She is now complaining of sensory loss along the upper medial thigh and weakness in the hip adductors.

Options for Questions 15–20

For each of the following clinical scenarios, choose the most appropriate diagnosis. Each option may be used once, more than once, or not at all.

A. Abruption
B. Acute asthma
C. Amniotic fluid embolism
D. Anaphylaxis
E. Diabetic ketoacidosis

F. Intracranial haemorrhage

G. Intracranial infarction

H. Placenta praevia

I. Puerperal psychosis

J. Pulmonary embolus

K. Pyelonephritis

L. Sepsis

M. Uterine inversion

N. Uterine rupture

15. A 26-year-old primigravid woman has an uncomplicated normal vaginal delivery. As the placenta is being delivered she suddenly collapses and becomes unresponsive. Her heart rate is 40 bpm and blood pressure is 50/30. The estimated blood loss is 200 ml.

16. A 35-year-old primigravid woman underwent induction of labour for post-dates with syntocinon augmentation. After a three-hour second stage she delivered a 4.2 kg baby but suddenly collapsed shortly after delivery.

17. A 42-year-old multiparous woman delivers a 1.5 kg baby using forceps at 36 weeks gestation. She has an active third stage. Forty minutes later she falls to one side and becomes unresponsive.

18. A 17-year-old woman delivers a healthy baby following induction of labour for prolonged rupture of membranes at 36 weeks gestation. She returns to casualty two weeks later complaining of palpitations and feeling generally unwell. Her observations are: heart rate 90 bpm, blood pressure 110/70. She is reassured and sent home. She later collapses at home.

19. A 22-year-old multiparous woman attends the labour ward after breaking her waters. She is known to be group B Streptococcus-positive and is given prophylactic antibiotics followed by syntocinon augmentation. She complained of sudden shortness of breath and becomes flushed and agitated before collapsing.

20. A 16-year-old primigravid woman attends A&E with acute onset of back pain at 26 weeks gestation. She is known to have a monochorionic twin pregnancy. She is tachycardic and hypotensive. Her abdomen is soft and there is no vaginal bleeding.

Options for Questions 21–25

For each of the following clinical scenarios, choose the most appropriate option. Each option may be used once, more than once, or not at all.

A. Acute pyelonephritis

B. Atorvastatin

C. Diabetic keto-acidosis

D. Diet

E. Folic acid

F. Gestational diabetes

G. Glibenclamide

H. Gliclazide

I. Impaired glucose tolerance

J. Insulin

K. Metformin

L. Ramipril

M. Steroids

N. Type 1 diabetes

O. Type 2 diabetes

P. Ultrasound

21. A 37-year-old white woman is referred to the antenatal clinic following an abnormal oral glucose tolerance test. She is 30 weeks pregnant with a symphysial fundal height of 34 cm, and an ultrasound scan reveals both abdominal circumference and liquor volume to be above the 95th centile. What is the best treatment option for this woman?

22. A healthy 28-year-old primigravid woman is referred to the antenatal clinic at 28 weeks pregnant to discuss her blood test results. Fasting blood glucose = 6.0 mmol/L and two hours after 75 g oral glucose tolerance test (OGTT) = 7.5 mmol/L. What is her diagnosis?

23. At pre-pregnancy counselling, a 32-year-old woman with type 1 diabetes comes to discuss optimizing her medications before conception. Which medication should be stopped to reduce the risk of limb deformities or CNS abnormalities?

24. A 30-year-old nulliparous insulin-dependent diabetic woman with a BMI of 49 is complaining of reduced foetal movements and feeling generally unwell. Her biochemistry shows bicarbonate levels below 10. What is the diagnosis?

25. A 34-year-old multiparous woman with a BMI of 40 has been diagnosed with gestational diabetes mellitus. She has noted reduced foetal movements and a drop in her insulin requirements over the past 24 hours. What is your management plan?

Options for Questions 26–30

The following questions concern shoulder dystocia. Choose the most appropriate *immediate* next course of action. Each option may be used once, more than once, or not at all.

A. Book elective caesarean section at 39–40 weeks

B. Book induction of labour at 39 weeks

C. Call for help

D. Cleidotomy

E. Deliver posterior arm

F. Discourage pushing, move buttocks to edge of the bed

G. Encourage pushing, move buttocks to edge of the bed

H. Episiotomy to aid delivery of the shoulders

I. Episiotomy to aid internal manoeuvres

J. Fundal pressure

K. Inform consultant obstetrician

L. Internal rotational manoeuvres

M. McRoberts' manoeuvre

N. Move patient into all-fours position

O. Suprapubic pressure

P. Symphysiotomy

Q. Zavanelli manoeuvre

26. A 38-year-old woman in her first pregnancy with gestational diabetes is seen at 37 weeks following a growth scan. The growth velocity is normal, with an estimated foetal weight of 4.8 kg, normal AFI, and normal Dopplers. She is keen for the safest mode of delivery for her baby.

27. A 27-year-old woman presents in her third pregnancy. Her second delivery was complicated by shoulder dystocia following a post-date induction of labour. The baby weighed 3.6 kg and is

fit and well now. Her old notes are not available but she recalls the midwives moving her legs and 'the baby came out'. She is now at 20 weeks and has not yet thought about the delivery of this baby.

28. You arrive in the labour ward room following the emergency buzzer. The midwife tells you she has diagnosed shoulder dystocia. The woman has an epidural and is in McRoberts' position, with the coordinator applying suprapubic pressure.

29. You pop your head into birthing unit room 3 as the junior midwife has called for assistance at her third delivery as a qualified midwife. The woman is just delivering and you notice that there was difficulty in delivering the head and the chin. There is no restitution. You pull the emergency buzzer for help.

30. You return from the gynaecology theatres and hear the emergency buzzer going off on the labour ward. On arrival you find a multiparous woman with no analgesia in the McRoberts' position, with a large episiotomy. Your junior obstetrician tells you that he has tried all of the internal manoeuvres as well as suprapubic pressure but the baby has not been delivered after three minutes. An obstetric emergency call has been put out.

Options for Questions 31–35

For each of the following clinical scenarios, choose the most appropriate option. Each option may be used once, more than once, or not at all.

A. Anorexia nervosa
B. Asherman's syndrome
C. Bulimia
D. Congenital adrenal hyperplasia
E. Craniopharingioma
F. Cushing syndrome
G. Diabetes insipidus
H. Diabetes mellitus
I. Hyperaldosteronism
J. Hyperthyroidism
K. Kallmann's syndrome
L. Pheochromocytoma
M. Polycystic ovarian syndrome
N. Premature ovarian failure
O. Prolactinoma
P. Sheehan's syndrome

31. A 31-year-old woman with a BMI of 22 presents with infertility of four years. She also complains of headaches, sweating, palpitations, and tremors. Her blood pressure is elevated during these episodes and the GP has attributed this to panic attacks.

32. A 26-year-old woman with a BMI of 23 presents with infertility of 24 months. She has occasional headaches and misses her periods sometimes. She is normotensive. Blood results are as follows: FSH 4, LH 6.4, prolactin 1790, TSH 3.4. Ultrasound shows multiple follicles and the largest measures 14 mm.

33. A 33-year-old multiparous woman underwent a normal vaginal delivery at 39 weeks gestation with her first pregnancy. She then experienced a delayed miscarriage with her subsequent pregnancy at eight weeks. She had surgical management of her miscarriage and was readmitted with abnormal discharge and fever a week later. Her periods are regular but she has only a day of very light spotting.

34. A 25-year-old woman has very infrequent periods since stopping Dianette (cyproterone acetate and ethinylestradiol) which was started at the age of 16 for acne. Her BMI is 31. She has declined a transvaginal ultrasound. Her day two hormone profile shows FSH 4, LH 8.3, prolactin 650.

35. A 30-year-old woman presents with a ten-month history of secondary amenorrhoea, feeling tired, and headaches. Her transvaginal ultrasound scan (TVUS) shows ovaries with antral follicle count (AFC) of 2 and normal uterus. Repeat investigations reveal FSH 42, LH 38, prolactin 150.

Options for Questions 36–40

Regarding antihypertensive treatment in pregnancy, choose the correct answer from the following list. Each option may be used once, more than once, or not at all.

  A. Admit to antenatal ward
  B. Atenolol
  C. Bed rest
  D. Bendroflumethiazide
  E. Doxazocin
  F. Enalapril
  G. Hydralazine im
  H. Hydralazine iv
  I. Labetalol im
  J. Labetalol iv
  K. Labetalol oral
  L. Low salt intake
  M. Methyldopa
  N. Monitor BP at home
  O. Nifedipine
  P. Ramipril

36. The first-line treatment for a 24-year-old asthmatic woman presenting with moderate hypertension (blood pressure 150/93) at 28 weeks of pregnancy.

37. The first-line drug for a 39-year-old primigravid woman diagnosed with pre-eclampsia and moderate hypertension at 32 weeks of pregnancy.

38. The most appropriate drug for a 34-year-old postnatal breastfeeding woman with renal disease who requires an ACE inhibitor for renal protection.

39. A 36-year-old woman on two medications for pre-eclampsia undergoes a normal vaginal delivery following induction of labour. Her blood pressure has been stable when taking medication. Which medication should now be stopped or changed postnatally?

40. A 22-year-old nulliparous woman at 30 weeks of pregnancy with blood pressure of 160/105 mmHg complains of upper abdominal discomfort and frontal headache.

Options for Questions 41–45

For each of the following clinical scenarios, choose the best initial investigation. Each answer may be used once, more than once, or not at all.

  A. Bladder diary
  B. Cystoscopy
  C. Hysteroscopy
  D. Intravenous pyelogram

    E. Laparoscopy

    F. Laparoscopy and cystoscopy

    G. Midstream urine

    H. MRI of pelvis

    I. Nerve studies

    J. Ultrasound

    K. Urine dipstick

    L. Urodynamics

41. A 36-year-old woman presents with urinary incontinence. She has some associated urinary frequency and some suprapubic pain.

42. A 47-year-old personal trainer presents with urinary leaking when weight training at the gym. She also needs to wear a sanitary towel due to some urge incontinence. Her GP has tried oxybutynin but to no avail. Her urine dipstick is normal.

43. A 35-year-old woman presents with a five-month history of suprapubic pain when passing urine. Urine dipstick persistently shows microscopic haematuria. Her urine cultures have not grown any organism.

44. A 40-year-old woman with menorrhagia attends the urogynaecology clinic with difficulty voiding. On examination, she has a 16-week-sized mass in her abdomen.

45. A 59-year-old para 6 woman presents with urinary incontinence and a mass in her vagina. She has tried pelvic floor exercises but they have not helped her symptoms.

Options for Questions 46–50

For each of the following clinical scenarios, choose the most appropriate treatment. Each option may be used once, more than once, or not at all.

    A. Cyclical hormone replacement therapy

    B. Cyclical progestogens

    C. Endometrial biopsy

    D. GnRH analogues

    E. Hysterectomy

    F. Insertion of levenorgestrel-containing IUS

    G. Iron treatment

    H. Laparoscopic myomectomy using morcellator

    I. MRI-guided focused ultrasound therapy

    J. Myomectomy

    K. Outpatient hysteroscopy and polypectomy

    L. Reassurance

    M. Transcervical resection of fibroid

    N. Uterine ablation

    O. Uterine artery embolization

46. A woman presents with heavy menstrual bleeding (HMB) and an enlarged uterus containing three separate intramural fibroids measuring 3–6 cm in diameter. She has had one previous child delivered by caesarean section and is 'pretty sure' she has completed her family. She does not want a major operation but requests permanent treatment.

47. The first-line treatment of HMB in a 44-year-old woman with multiple intramural fibroids within her uterine wall, the largest of which is 8 cm and a normal appearance to her endometrium.

48. A 29-year-old nulliparous woman with recurrent pelvic pressure symptoms and a single 8 cm pedunculated serosal fibroid that has been shown on MRI scan to be attached to the uterus by a 2 cm-thick pedicle.

49. A 48-year-old woman presents with HMB with a haemoglobin count of 79 g/L persistently despite regular iron therapy and medical treatment in the past. All investigations have been normal.

50. A 36-year-old nulliparous woman with a BMI of 25 is complaining of irregular periods for the past 12 months. Haemoglobin level is 10 g/dl. She had a previous large loop excision of her cervix. Pelvic ultrasound scan is normal.

Single Best Answers

1. D. Recruitment interview

Formative assessments inform learners of their progress and direct their learning, while summative assessments assess learning and contain decisions (pass/fail). Thus examples of formative assessments include induction interviews, team observation 1 forms, mini-clinical evaluation exercises, case-based discussion, and objective structured assessment of training. Examples of summative assessment include membership exams and ARCP outcomes. A recruitment interview allows you to demonstrate competence and is therefore an assessment of learning.

Parry-Smith W, Mahmud A, Landau A, Hayes K. WPBA: a new approach to existing tools. *TOG* 2014;16;281–85.

Shehmar M, Khan K. A guide to the ATSM in medical education. Article 2: Assessment, feedback and evaluation. *TOG* 2010;12:119–25.

2. E. 75%

Women with a RMI of less than 25 have a risk of cancer less than 3%. Women with a RMI between 25 and 250 have a 20% risk of cancer, and those with a RMI over 250 have a 75% risk of cancer.

RCOG Green-top Guideline 34. The management of ovarian cysts in post-menopausal women; 2016.

3. E. Respiratory distress syndrome

Of the options provided, this is the most commonly seen neonatal disorder in women with poorly controlled diabetes.

NICE Guideline NG3. Diabetes in pregnancy: management from preconception to the postnatal period; 2015, updated 2020.

4. C. Administer isoniazid and vitamin B6

If tuberculosis is diagnosed postnatally (sputum positive within two weeks of delivery) the disease may be transmitted to the newborn. Therefore prophylactic isoniazid and pyridoxine should be given. A tuberculin test should be performed at 6–12 weeks; if positive, the treatment should be continued for six months. If negative, medication can be stopped but the BCG vaccination should be given. Breastfeeding can be continued throughout.

Mahendru A, Gajjar K, Eddy J. Diagnosis and management of tuberculosis in pregnancy. *TOG* 2010;12:163–70.

5. A. Autologous blood transfusion

Jehovah's Witnesses do not accept the use of whole blood or blood components such as red cells, platelets, or plasma. Red cell salvage is accepted. It is important to adopt a lower threshold for medical and surgical management, including hysterectomy for women who decline blood.

Zeybek B, Childress AM, Kilic GS, Phelps JY, Pacheco LD, Carter MA, Borahay MA. Management of the Jehovah's Witness in obstetrics and gynecology: a comprehensive medical, ethical, and legal approach. *Obstet Gynecol Surv* 2016;71(8):488–500.

Blood Transfusion in Obstetrics

Nandi A, Gangopadhyay R. Management of women who decline blood and blood products in pregnancy. *TOG* 2010;12(2):138.

RCOG Green-top Guideline 47. Blood transfusion in obstetrics; May 2015.

6. A. Haemolytic anaemia

Laboratory investigations suggestive of congenital CMV infection include haemolytic anaemia, thrombocytopaenia, hepatitis, and hyperbilirubinaemia. Microcephaly is not a laboratory finding.

McCarthy F, Jones C, Rowlands S, Giles M. Primary and secondary cytomegalovirus in pregnancy. *TOG* 2009;11:96–100.

7. C. Pruritus

Two-thirds of women with VIN experience pruritus, while 20% remain asymptomatic.

Cullis P, Mudzamiri T, Millan D, Siddiqui N. Vulval intraepithelial neoplasia: making sense of the literature. *TOG* 2011;13:73–8.

RCOG and BGCS guidelines for the diagnosis and management of vulval carcinoma; 2014.

8. B. The levonorgestrel-releasing intrauterine system

Management of adenomyosis should be directed towards the symptoms experienced. Hysterectomy is not first-line management for adenomyosis.

Mehasseb M, et al. Adenomyosis uteri: an update. *TOG* 2009;11:1.

9. D. Reassure and discharge home

When a woman presents with vaginal spotting which has settled with no history of placenta praevia, she can be reassured and discharged. However, if the bleeding becomes heavier she should be admitted for observation at least until the bleeding stops.

RCOG Green-top Guideline 63. Antepartum haemorrhage; November 2011.

10. D. Total motility 40%

The WHO reference limits for semen parameters are as follows: semen volume 1.5 ml or more; sperm concentration 15×10^6/ml; total number of sperm 39×10^6/ml; total motility 40% (32% are progressive); normal forms 4%.

Karavolos S, Stewart J, Evbuomwan I, McEleny K, Aird I. Assessment of the infertile male. *TOG* 2013;15:1–9.

NICE Guidance. Fertility problems; 2014.

11. D. Reduction in the risk of colorectal cancer

The COCP protects against ovarian, endometrial, and colorectal cancer. It is also known to alleviate premenstrual syndrome. It can also be used to treat hirsutism and symptoms of polycystic ovary syndrome as well. A reduction in HMB and dysmenorrhoea is also seen.

Carey S, Allen R. Non-contraceptive uses and benefits of combined oral contraception. *TOG* 2012;14:223–8.

12. C. Perform a CTG

Basic assessment for women who present with reduced foetal movements include a detailed history, assessment of risk factors, maternal heart rate, blood pressure, temperature, urinalysis, CTG, and abdominal palpation. Women may be asked to lie on their left side to focus on foetal movements for 2 hours. Measurement of the amniotic fluid index and foetal biometry can then be performed.

RCOG Green-top Guideline 57. Reduced Fetal Movements, 2011.

Unterscheider J, Horgan R, O'Donoghue K, Greene R. Reduced fetal movements. *TOG* 2009;11:245–51.

13. E. An ultrasound should be performed to exclude endogenous oestrogen in women with atypical hyperplasia

In cases of simple or cystic hyperplasia, the malignant potential is so low that conservative management is appropriate. With atypical hyperplasia, there is a high rate of co-existing endometrial cancer and an even higher risk of the subsequent development of cancer. Thus TAH and BSO are the treatment of choice. In cases of adenomatous/complex hyperplasia, there is limited malignant potential. In this group, hysteroscopy will identify other endometrial pathology and allow further endometrial sampling. Sources of exogenous (e.g. tamoxifen) and endogenous (ovarian cancer) oestrogen should be excluded by history and examination/scanning. Treatment options for the simple and adenomatous groups are aimed at symptom control.

BSGE and RCOG Green-top Guideline 67. Management of endometrial hyperplasia; 2016.

Palmer J, Perunovic B, Tidy J. Endometrial hyperplasia. *TOG* 2011;10(4):211–16.

14. A. The 2020 MBRRACE-UK Perinatal Mortality Surveillance Report noted a 19% increase in twin stillbirth rate

In the UK, perinatal death is defined as the death of a foetus or a newborn in the perinatal period that commences at 24 completed weeks gestation and ends before seven completed days after birth. The traditionally used Wigglesworth and Aberdeen (obstetric) classifications have consistently classified more than 60–70% of stillbirths as unexplained. This has led to newer classifications, such as the new Centre for Maternal and Child Enquiries (CMACE) classifications, which have reduced the proportion of unexplained stillbirths to 15% and 23%, respectively. In the UK, intrapartum stillbirths contributed to 8.8% of the total number of stillbirths in 2008. Respiratory disorders were the major contributors, while birth trauma contributed to 0.2 neonatal deaths per 1,000 livebirths.

Åhman E, Zupan J. *Neonatal and perinatal mortality: country, regional and global estimates 2004.* Geneva: World Health Organization; 2007.

Centre for Maternal and Child Enquiries (CMACE). *Perinatal mortality 2008: United Kingdom.* London: CMACE; 2010.

MBRRACE-UK. *Perinatal Mortality Surveillance Report for births.* MBRRACE-UK; 2020.

15. D. Levonorgesterel-containing intrauterine system (IUS)

Ovulation inhibition is the main mode of action of all combined CHC. This includes the combined oral contraceptive pill (COC), combined transdermal patch (CTP), and CVR. The main mode of action of the levonorgestrel-containing IUS is progestogen-induced endometrial atrophy which prevents implantation. In addition, there are changes in the endometrial stroma, an increase in endometrial phagocytic cells, and reduced sperm penetration due to increased viscosity of the cervical mucus. Traditional POPs containing levonorgestrel, norethisterone, or ethynodiol diacetate mainly work by altering cervical mucus to prevent sperm penetration. There is also a variable degree of interference with ovulation; up to 60% of cycles may be anovulatory. In contrast, the primary mode of action of the desogestrel-containing POP (Cerazette®) is inhibition of ovulation (up to 97% of cycles). The primary mode of action for the subdermal implant is prevention of ovulation. In addition, cervical mucus is altered which prevents sperm penetration. Normal endometrial development is also inhibited which creates an unfavourable environment for implantation.

Faculty of Sexual & Reproductive Health (FSRH). Clinical Guideline: Intrauterine contraception. 2015, amended 2019.

FSRH Clinical Effectiveness Unit Clinical Guidance. Combined hormonal contraception. Progestogen-only pills. Injectable contraception. Subdermal implants. Intrauterine contraception; 2011.

16. B. Kleihauer test

Major foetal-maternal haemorrhage is a silent cause of IUD. Therefore a Kleihauer test is recommended for all women (not just Rhesus negative women). Ideally, blood tests should be taken before birth as foetal red cells may clear quickly from maternal circulation. Maternal coagulation times and plasma fibrinogen are not diagnostic tests for determining the cause of late IUD. However, they are important in the management of the patient. There is a risk of maternal disseminated intravascular coagulation (DIC): 10% within four weeks after the date of late IUD, rising to 30% thereafter. This can be tested for by clotting studies, platelet count, and fibrinogen measurement. Tests should be repeated twice weekly in women who choose expectant management. It is especially important to perform this test in case the patient would like regional anaesthesia during labour, which is contraindicated in the presence of abnormal coagulation. Placental pathology is useful and should be offered even if a post-mortem examination of the baby is declined. One review showed that in 88% of autopsy reports from stillbirths, examination of the placenta provided additional information to explain the cause of IUD. Medical imaging can act as an adjunct to full post-mortem. However, one study of perinatal deaths showed that if MRI were the only investigation, essential information would have been lost in 17% of cases. MRI is currently being evaluated further but is not yet suitable for clinical service. Skin specimens are associated with a higher rate of culture failure (60%), which is twice that of other tissues. A range of tissue types can be used but all cell cultures can fail. Therefore samples from multiple tissues should be used to increase the chance of culture.

Biankin SA, Arbuckle SM, Graf NS. Autopsy findings in a series of five cases of fetomaternal haemorrhages. *Pathology* 2003;35:319–24.

Cernach MC, Patricio FR, Galera MF, Moron AF, Brunoni D. Evaluation of a protocol for postmortem examination of stillbirths and neonatal deaths with congenital anomalies. *Pediatr Dev Pathol* 2004;7:335–41.

Kidron D, Bernheim J, Aviram R. Placental findings contributing to fetal death: a study of 120 stillbirths between 23 and 40 weeks gestation. *Placenta* 2009;30:700–4.

Parasnis H, Raje B, Hinduja IN. Relevance of plasma fibrinogen estimation in obstetric complications. *J Postgrad Med* 1992;38:183–5.

RCOG Green-top Guideline 55. Late intrauterine fetal death and stillbirth; 2010.

17. **E.** Spinal cord injury

Maternal indications to decrease the length and impact of the second stage of labour on medical conditions include hypertensive crises, significant cardiac disease, myasthenia gravis, proliferative retinopathy, and spinal cord injury patients who are at risk of autonomic dysreflexia.

ACOG Committee Opinion No 808. Obstetric management of patients with spinal cord injuries; 2020.

18. **D.** Selective oestrogen receptor modulator

Tamoxifen is a selective oestrogen receptor modulator (SERM). Although the primary therapeutic effect of tamoxifen is derived from its antiestrogenic properties, this agent also has modest oestrogenic activity and is associated with endometrial proliferation, hyperplasia, polyp formation, invasive carcinoma, and uterine sarcoma.

ACOG Committee Opinion No 601. Tamoxifen and uterine cancer; 2014.

19. **C.** Pre-eclampsia is a protective factor

Breast cancer affects 1 in 3,000 pregnant women. Risk factors for the development of breast cancer include nulliparity, early menarche, late first pregnancy, *BRCA1* and *BRCA2* mutations. The risk of breast cancer is also transiently increased after pregnancy for a maximum of 3–4 years. Protective factors include higher parity, pre-eclampsia, and hypertension in pregnancy. Breastfeeding is protective and related to duration.

Surgical excision can be undertaken at any stage in pregnancy but reconstruction should be delayed until after delivery to avoid prolonged anaesthesia. Chemotherapy should be avoided in the first trimester due to the high risk of foetal abnormality. Radiotherapy is contraindicated until delivery, unless lifesaving. Tamoxifen is contraindicated in pregnancy.

Breastfeeding from the contralateral normal breast is safe, but breastfeeding is contraindicated if taking tamoxifen or chemotherapy, as it is uncertain how much drug passes into the breast milk. A minimum of 14 days must elapse after completing chemotherapy before restarting breastfeeding.

The long-term survival after breast cancer is not adversely affected by pregnancy. Women should generally be advised to wait at least two years after treatment as the risk of cancer recurrence is highest in the early years.

RCOG Green-top Guideline 12. Pregnancy and breast cancer; 2011.

20. **C.** Nucleoside reverse transcriptase inhibitor

The three classes of antiretroviral drug most commonly used in pregnancy are nucleoside reverse transcriptase inhibitors (NRTI), non-nucleoside reverse transcriptase inhibitors (NNRTI), and protease inhibitors (PI). The most common regimens include a combination of two NRTI and a protease inhibitor or a non-nucleoside analogue. Treatment protocols are individualized for each patient. The safety and efficacy of the most common HAART regimens have not been studied in pregnancy. The BHIVA 2019 guidelines recommend starting with tenofovir and emtricitabine, or abacavir and lamivudine.

BHIVA Guideline. Management of HIV in pregnancy and postpartum; 2018.

21. C. Arrange serial growth scans

Isolated short femur length below the fifth or tenth centile may be an isolated finding at 20 weeks or it may be a marker for foetal growth restriction, preterm birth, and other adverse perinatal outcomes.

Goetzinger K, Cahill A, Macones G, Odibo A. Isolated short femur length on second trimester sonography. *J Ultrasound Med* 2012;31(12):1935–41.

22. B. IVF is more successful in women who have had a previous pregnancy

Smoking reduces the success rate in IVF cycles as it affects sperm function. US data has shown a reduced success rate if caffeine intake is high. Obesity affects the ovarian response to stimulation but obesity in the male also affects semen parameters. ICSI is a recognized method of treatment for oligozoospermia.

NICE Clinical Guideline 156. Assessment and treatment for people with fertility problems; 2013, updated 2017.

23. D. Tests such as rapid immunoassay AmniSure® have a specificity of 100% and sensitivity of 99%

Ultrasonographic detection of oligohydramnios helps to confirm the diagnosis of PPROM in the presence of a suggestive history and examination, but should not be used in isolation as oligohydramnios may be caused by other conditions such as placental insufficiency or foetal urinary tract abnormality. Tests such as the rapid immunoassay AmniSure® measures placental alpha macroglobulin-1 (PAMG-1) in vaginal fluid and has a sensitivity of 98.9% and specificity of 100%. Weekly high vaginal swabs have not been shown to increase the detection rate of chorioamnionitis. There is a risk of introducing infection by repeated examinations. Chorioamnionitis usually manifests as maternal pyrexia, offensive vaginal discharge, and foetal tachycardia. Blood tests for inflammatory markers, while helpful, are not necessarily accurate for the prediction of chorioamnionitis. The sensitivities of leucocytosis in the detection of clinical chorioamnionitis range from 29% to 47% and false positive rates from 5% to 18%, while the specificity of C-reactive protein is 38% to –55%. Chorioamnionitis is often subclinical with signs of infection such as pyrexia, uterine tenderness, and foul-smelling liquor present in only 30% of cases with proven microbial invasion.

Norman J, Greer I, eds. *Preterm labour: managing risk in clinical practice*. Cambridge: Cambridge University Press; 2005.

RCOG Green-top Guideline 73. Care of women presenting with suspected preterm prelabour rupture of membranes from 24 + 0 weeks of gestation; 2019.

24. B. Colposcopically directed punch biopsy should be performed if the transformational zone appears atypical

Cervical screening ends at 65 years. It begins at 25 years (in Scotland at 20 years). The screening interval is every three years between 25–49 years, and every five years between 50–64 years. In a recognizably atypical transformation zone, histological diagnosis must be available in all cases (100%). If routine cervical screening is due and the woman is pregnant, the test should be deferred. If the previous test is abnormal and she is now pregnant, referral to colposcopy should not be delayed.

NHS Cervical Screening Programme (NHSCSP) 20. May 2010, updated 2023.

25. B. It is safe to breastfeed while on propylthiouracil

Both PTU and carbimazole cross the placenta and, in a very high dose, may cause foetal hypothyroidism. One of the rare side effects of carbimazole is aplasia cutis. Beta blockers are used to treat tachycardia, sweating, and tremor. Radioactive iodine is contraindicated in pregnancy and breastfeeding since it is taken up by foetal thyroid. It is safe to breastfeed while on PTU.

Nelson-Piercy C. *Obstetric medicine*, 6th ed. Boca Raton: CRC Press; 2020.

26. C. Duloxetine

Duloxetine is licensed for use in stress incontinence. Its use should be reserved for cases refractory to conservative measures and where surgery is inappropriate. As this patient has ulcerative colitis, antimuscarinics should be avoided if possible.

NICE CKS. Incontinence: urinary, in women; 2019.

27. C. A 30-year-old woman with a history of painless miscarriage at 23 weeks

A history-induced cerclage should be offered following three preterm births or late (second-trimester) miscarriages. Without a history suggestive of cervical weakness (preterm delivery/late miscarriage), an incidental finding of cervical shortening is not an indication for cerclage insertion. History or ultrasound-induced cerclage is not recommended in multiple pregnancies—there is evidence to suggest that it may be detrimental, and is associated with both preterm delivery and pregnancy loss. A transabdominal cerclage may be used following extensive cervical surgery (e.g. radical trachelectomy) or when transvaginal cerclage has previously failed. The procedure is associated with increased maternal morbidity compared with transvaginal cerclage, and can be performed preconceptually or in early pregnancy. PPROM is a contraindication to cerclage insertion. Other contraindications include active preterm labour, evidence of chorioamnionitis, vaginal bleeding, foetal compromise, lethal foetal defect, and foetal death.

RCOG Green-top Guideline 75. Cervical cerclage; 2022, updated 2023.

28. D. Upon surgical evacuation, partial moles have foetal tissue or foetal red blood cells present

Molar pregnancies are either complete or partial moles based on their genetic and histopathological features. Complete moles are diploid and androgenic in origin, with no foetal tissue. Partial moles are usually (90%) triploid in origin, and primarily occur following dispermic fertilization of an ovum. In a partial mole, there is usually evidence of a foetus or foetal red blood cells. Asian women have a higher incidence of GTD compared with non-Asian women (1 in 387 vs. 1 in 752 live births). Although ultrasound is a key investigation in identifying a molar pregnancy, the diagnosis is a histological one. Women with GTD may be treated with chemotherapy, but radiotherapy is not required. The need for chemotherapy following a complete mole is 15% and 0.5% after a partial mole. Although surgical evacuation is the best modality of treatment, oxytocic infusions should not be used prior to completion of the evacuation. Anti-D should be administered to all women needing an evacuation.

RCOG Green-top Guideline 38. The management of gestational trophoblastic disease; February 2020.

29. B. The risk of twin stillbirth is over twice that of singletons

The recent MBRRACE-UK report noted that the risk of twin stillbirth is over 2.25 times higher than that of singletons. About one-third of twin pregnancies in the UK have monochorionic placenta. Monochorionic placentation can also occur in higher-order multiple pregnancies. Twin pregnancies are associated with increased risk of preterm births, foetal growth restriction, pre-eclampsia, maternal pregnancy symptoms, and post-partum haemorrhage. Monochorionic pregnancies are associated with vascular placental anatomies causing TTTS. TTTS complicates 10–15% of MC pregnancies. This leads to discordant growth. TTTS is more common in MCDA pregnancies than

MCMA pregnancies. Significant discordant growth can also occur in MC twins in the absence of TTTS in approximately 10% of pregnancies.

Kilby M, et al. *Multiple pregnancy.* London: RCOG Press; 2006.

MBRRACE-UK Perinatal Mortality Surveillance Report for births; 2020.

Quintero RAM. Stage-based treatment of twin-twin transfusion syndrome. *Am J Obstet Gynecol* 2003;188:1333–40.

RCOG Green-top Guideline 51. Management of monochorionic twin pregnancy; 2016.

30. E. Recurrent episodes of genital herpes is associated with a 3% risk of neonatal herpes, even if lesions are present at the time of delivery

Local central nervous system disease (encephalitis alone), one of the subgroups of neonatal herpes, often presents late, and is associated with a mortality rate of 6% and neurological morbidity of 70% if treated. The most common route of transmission of the virus is by contact with infected maternal secretions. The risk of transmission of HSV to the foetus during a vaginal delivery in a woman with a history of recurrent genital herpes is 1–3% and vaginal delivery is not contraindicated in the absence of other obstetric indications for caesarean section. Foetal scalp electrodes and foetal blood sampling in labour are to be avoided in women with recurrent genital herpes, even though she has not had a recurrence in labour.

BASH/RCOG. Management of genital herpes in pregnancy; 2014.

31. B. Granulosa cell tumours

Granulosa theca cell tumours from the ovaries produce oestrogen. This does not respond to hypothalamic feedback, thus leading to high circulating levels of oestrogen. This unopposed oestrogen can stimulate the endometrium and lead to endometrial cancer.

NICE Clinical Guideline 122. Ovarian cancer: the recognition and initial management of ovarian cancer; 2011.

32. B. Hyponatraemia

Moderate OHSS is classed as moderate abdominal pain, ultrasound evidence of ascites, and ovarian size 8–12 cm. The severe form of OHSS is associated with clinical ascites and compromised renal function, as more fluid shifts from the intravascular to extravascular compartment, leading to reduced renal perfusion and oliguria, a haematocrit of >45%, and ovarian size more than 12 cm. When a patient presents with the foregoing signs and symptoms, she should be managed as an inpatient and reviewed daily to assess her condition. Critical OHSS is associated with tense ascites, haematocrit more than 55%, more extravascular fluid and compromised systemic function. An increase in WBC >25,000/ml indicates an ongoing systemic stress response. There is an increased risk of thromboembolism, acute renal failure, and ARDS, although ARDS and acute renal shutdown are very rare. Hyponatraemia is observed in 56% of cases and may be dilutional due to hypersecretion of antidiuretic hormone. Abnormal LFTs in 25–40% of cases resolve with the disease.

RCOG Green-top Guideline 5. Ovarian hyperstimulation syndrome; 2016.

33. A. The age-related risk of miscarriage in women over the age of 45 is over 90%

Recurrent miscarriage (loss of three or more consecutive pregnancies) affects 1% of couples. The age-related risk of miscarriage increases from 11% at 20–24 years, up to 93% in the over-45s population. Advancing paternal age is a risk factor for miscarriage. The risk of miscarriage is highest in a couple when the woman is 35 or older and her partner 40 or over. Antiphospholipid antibodies are present in 15% of women with recurrent miscarriage. The prevalence in women with low obstetric risk is 2%. If antiphospholipid antibodies are present, the live birth rate without pharmacological intervention may be as low as 10%.

Preimplantation genetic diagnosis (PIGD), plus the necessary IVF, has been proposed as a method to select genetically normal embryos. However, the live birth rate in women who conceive spontaneously is higher than that after PIGD and IVF.

RCOG Green-top Guideline 17. The investigation and treatment of couples with recurrent first-trimester and second-trimester miscarriage; 2011.

34. D. Non-immune hydrops

Sequelae of foetal infection associated with parvovirus B19 infection include miscarriage, anaemia, non-immune hydrops, and intrauterine death.

To M, Kidd M, Maxwell D. Prenatal diagnosis and management of fetal infections. *TOG* 2009;11:108–16.

35. B. 15%

This may be due to pre-existing detrusor overactivity which was subclinical until the surgery, or due to damage to the autonomic nerve supply to the bladder, which may be disrupted as the bladder is displaced medially during surgery.

BSUG. Colposuspension for Stress Urinary Incontinence: Patient information leaflet; 2018.

36. A. Amitryptiline

Treatment for vulvodynia includes local anaesthesia, amitriptyline and, later on, gabapentin. Other modes which may provide additional help include cognitive behaviour therapy and pelvic floor biofeedback.

BASHH UK National Guideline on the Management of Vulval Conditions; 2014.

37. A. She should be offered HIV testing of older children if their HIV status is unknown

Sexual health screening is also recommended for pregnant women who are newly diagnosed with HIV.

BHIVA. Guidelines for the management of HIV in pregnant women; 2012.

38. A. Estimated foetal weight below the tenth centile

Factors regarded as unfavourable for vaginal breech delivery include a footling or kneeling breech presentation, a large baby (EFW >3.8 kg) or a small baby (EFW <2 kg), hyperextended neck in labour, previous caesarean section, and the lack of a clinician trained in vaginal breech delivery. Other contraindications to vaginal delivery (e.g. placenta praevia) should also be considered.

NICE and National Guideline Alliance NG201. Antenatal care: management of breech presentation; 2021.

RCOG Green-top Guideline 20b. Management of the term breech; 2017.

39. E. Stab wounds are injuries that are deeper than they are long and have sharp wound edges

The injury described in option A is petechiae. An ecchymosis is a subcutaneous purpura measuring more than 1 cm. It is not caused by trauma. The injury described in option B is a bruise. Erythema is a redness of the skin caused by hyperaemia of the capillaries in the lower layers of the skin. It may occur with any skin injury, infection, or inflammation. The injury described in option C is an abrasion. Lacerations are characterized by damage to the skin and may involve the subcutaneous and muscular layers. The injury shows an irregular contour, bruising to the edges, and tissue strands such as nerves and fibrous bands crossing in the depth of the wound. The injury described in option D is a laceration. Lacerations may be caused by a variety of mechanisms. Slash wounds are incised wounds caused by a sharp cutting instrument, such as a knife. They are broader than they are deep. Another type of incised wound is a stab wound.

Knight B. Examination of wounds. In: Knight B, Simpson K (eds) *Simpson's forensic medicine.* Oxford: Oxford University Press; 1991, pp. 115–70.

Wyatt J, Squires T, Norfolk G, Payne-James J. *Forensic pathology of physical injury.* Oxford: Oxford Academic; 2011.

40. C. Mature cystic teratoma

The diagnosis here is ovarian cyst torsion, which is most commonly associated with mature dermoid cysts. Between 80–85% of mature cystic teratomas are unilateral, with a 1% malignancy rate. Solid structures within dermoid cysts include teeth enamel, hair, and sebum.

NICE Guideline 122. Ovarian cancer; 2011, updated 2017, 2021.

41. D. It should only be used once in a menstrual cycle

Ulipristal acetate (UPA) is a progesterone receptor modulator. The primary mechanism of action is thought to be inhibition or delay of ovulation. If administered immediately before ovulation, the growth of lead follicles is suppressed. There is some evidence that UPA can also prevent ovulation after the LH surge has started, delaying follicular rupture. Administration of UPA at the time of the LH peak or after does not appear to be effective in delaying follicular rupture. Although some studies have shown an endometrial effect, it is not known yet whether this can inhibit implantation.

Both UPA and levonorgestrel can be used as oral emergency contraception more than once in the same cycle. The summary of product characteristics (SPC) states that it is not advisable to use UPA with liver enzyme-inducing drugs. The Clinical Effectiveness Unit (CEU) of the Faculty of Sexual & Reproductive Health (FRSH) supports this advice. The CEU does not currently support doubling the dose of UPA when using drugs that may reduce UPA's efficacy.

Antacids, proton pump inhibitors, and H_2 receptor antagonists—and any other drugs that increase gastric pH—may reduce the absorption of UPA and decrease its efficacy. They should therefore not be used concomitantly.

There is no data on the efficacy or safety of using UPA outside the treatment window (>120 hours). The CEU of the FSRH does not currently support the use of UPA beyond 120 hours.

FSRH. New product review: ulipristal acetate; Oct. 2009.

Faculty of Sexual & Reproductive Health (FSRH) Clinical Effectiveness Unit (CEU) Guidance. Emergency contraception; 2017 (updated Dec 2020).

42. B. Multilocular cyst

The ultrasound features which contribute to the RMI include a multilocular cyst, bilateral lesion, evidence of solid areas within the cyst, evidence of metastases and the presence of ascites.

RCOG Green-top Guideline 34. Ovarian cysts in post-menopausal women; 2016.

43. C. Laparoscopic incision of endometriomas with drainage and irrigation is associated with low morbidity but more pain recurrence than excision

Medical treatment of laparoscopically diagnosed endometriosis does not improve the likelihood of conception. Surgical excision of mild to moderate endometriosis has superior outcomes in comparison to other treatment modalities regarding cyst recurrence, pain symptoms, and subsequent spontaneous pregnancy. Endometriosis is a progressive condition in more than 50% of cases. Cases of severe endometriosis should be managed within a multidisciplinary setting.

Hart R, et al. Excisional surgery versus ablative surgery for ovarian endometriomata. *Cochrane Database Syst Rev* 2008;2:1–31.

Prasannan-Nair C, Manias T, Mathur R. Management of endometriosis-related subfertility. *TOG* 2011;13(1):1–6.

44. C. Stress urinary incontinence

The involuntary leakage of urine without detrusor activity leads to a diagnosis of stress urinary incontinence.

NICE Clinical Guideline 123. Urinary incontinence and pelvic organ prolapse in women: the management; 2019.

45. D. Thrombotic thrombocytopaenic purpura

Thrombotic thrombocytopaenic purpura—also known as haemolytic uraemic syndrome—is a rare disorder which presents with haemolytic anaemia, thrombocytopaenia, neurological symptoms, renal dysfunction, and fever. It is due to a deficiency of von Willebrand's factor-cleaving protein (ADAMTS 13).

BMJ Best Practice. Thrombotic thrombocytopaenic purpura; 2022.

Myers B. Thrombocytopenia in pregnancy. *TOG* 2009;11:177–83.

46. C. Progestogen-only contraception can be started immediately after a first- or second-trimester termination of pregnancy

There is no evidence that progestogen-only pills, injectable contraception, implants, or the levonorgestrel-releasing intrauterine system are associated with an increased risk of venous thromboembolism. For women with current venous thromboembolism on anticoagulants or previous venous thromboembolism, progestogen-only contraception is safe. Women with factor V Leiden can have up to a 35-fold increase in the risk of VTE with COC use. For women who are post-partum and not breastfeeding, combined hormonal contraception (pill, patch, or vaginal ring) should be considered after day 21 post-partum only. All hormonal contraception can be safely initiated immediately following a first- or second-trimester termination of pregnancy.

Thrombosis UK. Thrombosis and women: periods, the contraceptive pill and HRT.

47. D. HPV subtypes 16 and 18 are associated with the development of cervical cancer

HPV is the most important risk factor for the development of cervical cancer. Smoking and poor socioeconomic status are also risk factors. 1A tumours are microscopic and not visible to the naked eye, whereas 1B tumours are always visible. 1B2 cervical cancers are defined as being at least 4 cm in their largest diameter, but confined to the cervix, and are therefore visible on examination. There are over 100 types of HPV; 16 and 18 are high-risk types for the development of cervical cancer. Types 6 and 11 are the HPV types associated with the development of genital warts. Squamous carcinoma is the most common histological subtype. Although adenocarcinoma typically presents at a more advanced stage, survival is approximately equivalent to squamous cancer of the same stage. Neither subtype of cervical cancer is thought to be hormone-dependent; therefore, it is largely accepted that surgical treatment of premenopausal women should include conservation of the ovaries. This prevents the cardiovascular and skeletal complications of premature menopause. Adenocarcinoma has been reported to metastasize to the ovaries, so careful inspection during surgery should be performed.

FIGO. Staging classification and clinical practice guidelines of gynaecologic cancers; 2003.

48. B. The need for repeat surgical evacuation after surgical management of miscarriage (SMM) is up to almost 20 in 1,000 women

A complication which occurs less than 1 in 10,000 is very rare. A frequent risk of surgical evacuation of the uterus is localized pelvic infection. Non-surgical methods are associated with up to a 50% possibility of eventually needing surgical evacuation. Non-surgical methods are associated with a lower risk of infection compared to surgical evacuation of the uterus.

RCOG Clinical Governance Advice 7. Presenting information on risk; 2008.

RCOG Consent Advice 10. Surgical management of miscarriage and removal of persistent placental or fetal remains; 2018.

49. E. Labour augmentation with syntocinon may be considered

Vaginal breech birth should occur in a hospital with the facilities for an emergency caesarean section together with an experienced clinician who is able to perform a breech delivery. Labour induction may be considered if favourable. Epidural analgesia is not routinely advised, **but** augmentation of slow progress with oxytocin may be considered if the contraction frequency is low in the presence of epidural analgesia. Breech extraction should not be used routinely and episiotomy should be performed when clinically indicated to facilitate delivery.

BJOG RCOG Green-top Guideline 20b. Management of the term breech; 2017: e151–77.

NICE and National Guideline Alliance NG201. Antenatal care: management of breech presentation; 2021.

50. B. Micturating cystourethroscopy

This is the most reliable way of detecting a fistula. Vesico-vaginal fistula is a rare complication. MRI and CT scans can show anatomical landmarks but they are not dynamic tests to show a urinary leak. A micturating cystourethroscopy will clearly demonstrate the track of the urine leak in the vaginal canal. It can also help to differentiate between a ureteric and bladder fistula into the vaginal canal.

StratOG: The RCOG online learning. Management of postoperative complications; investigation of the renal tract. Available at: https://www.rcog.org.uk

Extended Matching Questions

Answers for Questions 1–5

1. A; 2. D; 3. G; 4. H; 5. M

1. Risk of miscarriage is the lowest in the younger age group. Advanced maternal age and a previous history of recurrent miscarriage (>3) are independent risk factors. Advanced maternal age increases risks related to chromosomally abnormal pregnancies. Obesity is an independent risk factor, as the risk of spontaneous miscarriage incrementally increases with BMI.

2. The risk of a spontaneous miscarriage increases with advancing maternal age. There is a marginally increased risk of pregnancies being affected by trisomies; hence a spontaneous miscarriage may be part of natural selection.

3. Previous reproductive performance is an independent predictor of a miscarriage. Previous normal births are a positive predictor, whereas the risk of a further miscarriage increases after each successive pregnancy loss, approaching 40% after three consecutive pregnancy losses. Other factors, such as X-linked recessive traits, positive lupus anticoagulants, and maternal thrombosis, are also small contributions, as is the male partner's age (>40).

4. Maternal age is an independent risk factor for miscarriage and it relates to chromosomally abnormal fertilized oocytes. A male partner aged over 40, balanced chromosomal rearrangement, obesity, and lupus-positive screening also increase the risk of a miscarriage.

5. Maternal age is an independent risk factor for miscarriage and foetal aneuploidy is quite common in this age group. A higher incidence of pregnancies affected by trisomies and miscarriage is one way that nature selects potentially nonviable pregnancies. Environmental factors such as increased caffeine intake and cigarette smoking may have a dose-dependent effect, but there are insufficient data to confirm an association.

RCOG Green-top Guideline 17. Recurrent miscarriage: investigations and treatment of couples; 2011.

Answers for Questions 6–9

6. B; 7. I; 8. K; 9. D

6. Non-steroidal anti-inflammatory drugs should be avoided due to the potential impact on renal function.

7. Hypertonic saline should be administered as there is evidence of hyponatraemia. If her sodium was normal then normal saline could be used. Hartmann's solution should not be used as it contains potassium.

8. The most recent publications suggest that metformin is the drug of choice, although in some cases, bromocriptine has also been used.

9. GnRH antagonist regimens are associated with a decreased incidence of OHSS when compared with agonist regimens.

RCOG Green-top Guideline 5. The management of ovarian hyperstimulation syndrome; 2006, 3rd ed., 2016.

Answers for Questions 10–14

10. B; 11. D; 12. C; 13. H; 14. G

10. Femoral neuropathy commonly occurs as a result of compression of the nerve against the pelvic side wall as it emerges from the lateral border of the psoas muscle. This happens when deep retractor blades are used during the lateral placement of self-retaining retractors

for difficult operations. It can also occur when female patients are positioned inappropriately in lithotomy position.

11. Ileo-inguinal and ileo-hypogastric nerve damage is typically caused by the suture entrapment at the lateral border of lower transverse incision that has extended beyond the lateral border of the rectus abdominus muscle. Laparoscopic and retropubic midurethral tape procedures may also injure these nerves.

12. The genito-femoral nerve crosses the anterior surface of psoas muscle and lies lateral to the external iliac vessels. This nerve is susceptible to injury during pelvic side wall surgery and during removal of the external iliac lymph nodes.

13. The pudendal nerve (S2–4) exits the pelvis through the greater sciatic foramen and runs behind the lateral third of the sacrospinus ligament and ischial spine. The nerve is susceptible to entrapment during sacrospinus ligament fixation.

14. The obturator nerve (L2–4) passes over the pelvic brim in front of the sacroiliac joint. This nerve then passes over the pelvic rim in front of the sacroiliac joint and enters the thigh via the obturator foramen. The nerve is susceptible to injury during retroperitoneal surgery, excision of endometriosis, the passage of a trocar through obturator foramen and insertion of transobturator tape.

Kuponiyi O, et al. Nerve injuries associated with gynecological surgery. *TOG* 2014;16:29–36.

Answers for Questions 15–20

15. M; 16. N; 17. G; 18. L; 19. D; 20. A

15. This scenario describes profound shock that is not in keeping with the volume of blood lost. Collapse occurs with delivery of the placenta which suggests the possibility of uterine inversion.

16. There are a number of risk factors for PPH in this scenario but there is no mention of bleeding. The risk factors mentioned are also risk factors for uterine rupture which often causes intra-abdominal bleeding.

17. The most important features of this scenario are the growth-restricted baby being delivered early and the collapse to the side. The woman is age 42 and the link between increased maternal age and IUGR is pre-eclampsia. Syntometrine is the standard management for the third stage. This can cause hypertension, particularly if there is an underlying hypertensive disorder. Severe hypertension can result in intracranial hypertension and haemorrhage.

18. Sepsis is a growing problem in the obstetric population and is a significant cause of maternal morbidity and mortality. Prolonged SROM is a risk factor for sepsis and initial symptoms are often vague. In a young, normally healthy woman, an HR of 90 bpm is likely to be significant. It is also important to remember that young healthy women can maintain their observations until extreme cardiovascular compromise is reached.

19. The acute onset of shortness of breath with associated facial flushing and agitation reflects an anaphylactic reaction, most probably due to penicillin administered for the GBS infection. Other features of anaphylaxis include wheeze, itch, oedema, and stridor.

20. Abruption should always be part of the differential diagnosis when there is pain in pregnancy. Back pain can predominate if the placenta is posterior. Bleeding may be concealed or revealed and absence of vaginal bleeding does not exclude the diagnosis.

RCOG Green-top Guideline 56. Maternal collapse in pregnancy and the puerperium; 2011, updated 2019.

Answers for Questions 21–25

21. J; 22. F; 23. B; 24. C; 25. P

21. This woman already has signs of macrosomia and polyhydramnios, and prompt control of her blood sugars is necessary to reduce her risk of developing further complications. Most women with gestational diabetes mellitus (GDM) can be managed by altering their diet but 20–40% will require insulin therapy at some point in the pregnancy.

22. The definition of GDM is based on a 75 g two-hour OGTT. GDM is diagnosed if the woman has either fasting venous blood glucose ≥5.6 mmol/L, or a two-hour value ≥7.8 mmol/L.

23. Statins are contraindicated in pregnancy as there have been reports of unilateral limb deformities and CNS abnormalities, including holoprosencephaly.

24. Here, the history is suggestive of poorly controlled diabetes during pregnancy which obese women are more susceptible to. Low bicarbonate levels are suggestive of diabetic ketoacidosis.

25. A sudden reduction in insulin dosage and reduced foetal movements suggests failing placental function. Such women require urgent assessment of foetal well-being and of placental function. They are at increased risk of sudden foetal demise.

RCOG SAC Opinion Paper. Diagnosis and treatment of gestational diabetes; 2011, replaced by NICE NG 3: Diabetes in pregnancy: management from preconception to the postnatal period 2015, updated 2020.

Answers for Questions 26–30

26. A; 27. K28. H; 29. F; 30. N

26. An estimated foetal weight over 4.5 kg is an indication for an elective caesarean section due to the high risk of shoulder dystocia.

27. A full review of the notes needs to be undertaken if possible, and may require writing to the previous consultant in charge of her care. Following this, a full consultation needs to take place and then the mode of delivery can be confirmed at 36 weeks. A growth scan may be indicated at this point.

28. Considering the need for an episiotomy is the next stage in the HELPER mnemonic for delivery of shoulder dystocia.

29. The next step is to open the pelvis, either by McRoberts' manoeuvre or, as in this case (birthing room, no help), move the patient to the edge of the bed.

30. This is the next stage in the HELPER mnemonic.

RCOG Green-top Guideline 42. Shoulder dystocia; 2012.

Answers for Questions 31–35

31. L; 32. O; 33. B; 34. M; 35. N

31. The characteristics of a phaeochromocytoma include intermittent symptoms with an associated raised BP.

32. The diagnosis of a prolactinoma is confirmed by the presence of an elevated prolactin level.

33. Asherman's syndrome is likely with a regular but light period with a past history suggestive of infection.

34. Polycystic ovary syndrome is diagnosed according to the Rotterdam consensus definition, characterized here by the reversed LH/FSH ratio and irregular periods.

The Rotterdam criteria includes polycystic ovaries (12 or more follicle or increased ovarian volume over 10cc), oligo- or anovulation, clinical, and/or biochemical signs of hyperandrogenism.

35. Premature ovarian failure is the diagnosis given the reduced AFC and raised FSH; diagnosis is based on a combination of oligomenorrhoea/amenorrhoea of over 4 months duration with elevated FSH >40 on at least two occasions measured 4–6 weeks apart in women under the age of 40.

BMS Consensus Statement. Premature menopause; 2007, updated premature ovarian insufficiency; 2020.

RCOG Green-top Guideline 33. Long-term consequences of polycystic ovarian syndrome; 2014.

Answers for Questions 36–40

36. O; 37. K; 38. F; 39. M; 40. J

36. The 2019 NICE Guideline recommends labetalol as first-line therapy in pregnancy. However, the woman has asthma, so nifedipine is the recommended alternative.

37. As there is no history of asthma, labetalol is the first-choice antihypertensive agent.

38. There is limited information on the safety of most ACE inhibitors in breastfeeding. However, both captopril and enalapril are recommended by NICE for use in breastfeeding.

39. Methyldopa is associated with postnatal depression and should be stopped or replaced within 48 hours of delivery.

40. This is a case of severe pre-eclampsia and the first step is to control her blood pressure.

NICE Clinical Guideline 107, 133. Hypertension in pregnancy: diagnosis in pregnancy; 2010, updated 2019.

Answers for Questions 41–45

41. K; 42. L; 43. B; 44. J; 45. L

41. It is important to rule out a urinary tract infection first.

42. Mixed symptoms of urinary incontinence may not respond to primary care treatment of urge incontinence.

43. Cystoscopy should be considered in view of persistent haematuria.

44. It is important to investigate the nature of pelvic mass. Considering her symptoms of menorrhagia, it is possible that pressure symptoms from fibroids or an ovarian cyst are causing voiding difficulties.

45. The most likely cause is that she has a significant cystocele and would need an anterior repair and TVT.

NICE Guideline 174, 171. Urinary incontinence in women: Management; 2013, updated 2015.

Answers for Questions 46–50

46. O; 47. F; 48. J; 49. N; 50. B

46. Embolization is the most likely treatment with the potential for the lowest impact based on her requirements. The newer procedure of MRI-guided focused ultrasound would not be suitable as it is not yet fully researched and is contraindicated in those who have abdominal scars.

47. The levonorgestrel-containing intrauterine system would be the first-line treatment as per NICE guidance.

48. Open myomectomy is likely to be the safest option; morcellators are currently under review in the market. Embolization is not suitable for pedunculated serosal fibroids.

49. Endometrial ablation should be offered as first-line therapy in women with dysfunctional bleeding with normal investigations.

50. Although the levonorgestrel-containing IUS should be the first choice, it may not be possible to insert it in a nulliparous patient, particularly given the previous history of large loop excision, so cyclical progestogens or the COCP should be considered.

NICE Clinical Guideline 88. Heavy menstrual bleeding: assessment and management; 2018, updated 2021.

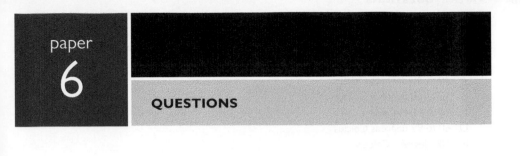
Single Best Answers

1. **Through what mechanism can surgical diathermy cause the thermal destruction of tissues?**
   A. Coagulation
   B. Dehumidification
   C. Haemolysis
   D. Hydration
   E. Vaporization

2. **Which one of the following is a branch of the inferior mesenteric artery?**
   A. Ileocolic artery
   B. Jejunal artery
   C. Left colic artery
   D. Ovarian artery
   E. Right colic artery

3. **Who one of the following is the definition for late neonatal death?**
   A. Death in the first 3 days of life
   B. Death in the first 6 days of life
   C. Death from age 4 days to 27 completed days of life
   D. Death from age 7 days to 27 completed days of life
   E. Death from 28 days to 3 completed months of life

4. **Which one of the following has a purine amino acid DNA base?**
   A. Adenine
   B. Alanine
   C. Arginine
   D. Asparagine
   E. Aspartic acid

5. **At what temperature generated through diathermy during surgery does coagulation occur?**
   A. 30 to 40 degrees Celcius
   B. 40 to 60 degrees Celcius
   C. 60 degrees Celcius
   D. 60 to 99 degrees Celcius
   E. 100 degrees Celcius

6. **Which one of the following is present in the deep perineal pouch?**
   A. Bulbs of the vestibules
   B. Bulbospongiosus
   C. Deep transverse perineal muscles
   D. Greater vestibular glands
   E. Superficial transverse perineal muscle

7. **Which of these energy forms in diathermy causes coagulation?**
   A. Continuous waveforms
   B. Continuous waveforms with low voltage
   C. Continuous waveforms with high voltage
   D. Pulsed waveform with low voltage
   E. Pulsed waveform with high voltage

8. **After a vasectomy for male sterilization, what is the incidence rate for chronic post-vasectomy pain?**
   A. 1%
   B. 1–14%
   C. 15–20%
   D. 25%
   E. 30–40%

9. **What is the 10-year cumulative probability of an ectopic pregnancy after a laparoscopic tubal sterilization?**
   A. 1.2–2.4 per 1,000 procedures
   B. 2.4–7.3 per 1,000 procedures
   C. 8.4–9.3 per 1,000 procedures
   D. 10.1–13.4 per 1,000 procedures
   E. 12.2–15.3 per 1,000 procedures

10. **You are the senior registrar on-call at night in a 3-tier unit. Your junior registrar is performing a caesarean section with the SHO, and they have just delivered the baby. You have examined a patient who has been pushing for 1 hour with no signs of imminent delivery and a suspicious CTG trace. You decide she needs a trial in theatre. There are two other ongoing labourers on IV oxytocin and a patient with placenta praevia has just arrived, with some vaginal bleeding. What is your next step?**
    A. Ask your patient to stop pushing.
    B. Call the theatre team, a second anaesthetist, and transfer the patient to theatre.
    C. Speak to the midwife co-ordinator about the situation and call your consultant.
    D. Stop the IV oxytocin of the other two labourers.
    E. Try and complete an instrumental in the room.

11. **You are working on a busy gynaecology ward. Your shift was meant to finish at 5pm but it is 7pm and you are still trying to complete some of your routine tasks from the day. This has happened a few times before and as a result you feel exhausted. Your workload is also having a negative impact on your social and family life. Your colleagues have advised you to exception report. What is the most important consideration for exception reporting?**
    A. The impact on your well-being if you do not have a social life.
    B. The risk to patient safety if working while tired.
    C. To ensure all tasks, even if not urgent, are completed on the day.
    D. Your right to finish at the designated time.
    E. Your consultant may give you a poor reference if you exemption report.

12. **The perineal body is formed of which of the following muscles?**
    A. Gluteus maximus
    B. Internal anal sphincter
    C. Ischiocavernous muscle
    D. Levator ani
    E. Levator ani and external anal sphincter

13. **A 16-year-old girl presents to the gynaecology clinic with delayed puberty, excessive facial hair, and on examination an enlarged clitoris. Tests show a low sodium and raised potassium level. An ultimate diagnosis of congenital adrenal hyperplasia is made. Which one of the following is the most common defect in the congenital adrenal hyperplasia (CAH)?**
    A. Defect in 3βHSD
    B. Defect in 5α-reductase
    C. Defect in 11β-hydroxylase
    D. Defect in 17α-hydroxylase
    E. Defect in 21α-hydroxylase

14. Which ONE of the following vitamin deficiencies causes Beriberi disease?

   A. Ascorbic acid

   B. Calciferol

   C. Folic acid

   D. Riboflavin

   E. Thiamine

15. In organ transplantation, which host versus graft rejection response commonly occurs within 10 days of procedure?

   A. Acute

   B. Acute early

   C. Acute late

   D. Chronic

   E. Hyperacute

16. You are the junior registrar on a night-shift and have just delivered a baby via ventouse delivery, with an episiotomy in the room. You have delivered the placenta and, while suturing, note that the bleeding is ongoing and reaching an estimated blood loss of 850 ml. She has a working epidural. What would your next step be?

   A. Assess the basics; airway, breathing, circulation (ABC). As she is stable you continue suturing.

   B. After ABC, call for help while assessing if the bleeding is caused by trauma, tissue, tone, thrombus (4Ts).

   C. Continue to suture as you believe the bleeding is caused by trauma.

   D. Stop suturing and check the tone of the uterus.

   E. The patient is stable, but the bleeding is ongoing, so pull the emergency buzzer and take the patient to theatre.

17. What does the communication tool acronym SBAR stand for?

   A. Situation, background, assessment, recommendation

   B. Significance, background, assessment, recommendation

   C. Situation, background, action, recommendation

   D. Significance, background, action, report

   E. Situation, background, assessment, report

18. You are an ST5 trainee about to progress to ST6. You have just had your ARCP and received an outcome 3. Which of the following best explains this outcome?

   A. Development of specific competences required—additional training time not required

   B. Inadequate progress—additional training time required

   C. Incomplete evidence presented—additional training time may be required

   D. Released from the training programme—without specific competencies

   E. Satisfactory progress—achieving progress and the development of competences at the expected rate.

19. **A GP trainee working in obstetrics and gynaecology has asked you to complete an assessment for performing a smear test. You observe him performing the procedure and agree to sign his assessment form. Which of the following workplace-based assessment is best suited for this assessment?**

A. ARCP

B. CBD

C. DOPS

D. Mini-CEX

E. TO1

20. **Preet is approaching the end of ST5 and is keen to apply for gynaecology oncology subspeciality training. However, she has never heard of an Asian doctor successfully attaining this role. As a result she continues with her training, shelving her desires in order to avoid being unsuccessful in getting the role to subspecialize. Which of the following levels of racism is described here?**

A. Internalized racism

B. Interpersonal racism

C. Direct discrimination

D. Discrimination by association

E. Systemic racism

21. **You have been called to assess a 28-year-old woman in spontaneous labour who has been pushing for 1 hour. She has had previously had one normal vaginal delivery. Abdominal examination confirms 1/5 palpable per abdomen. Vaginal examination confirms she is fully dilated, cephalic presentation, with the presenting part at the ischial spines, anterior fontanelle palpable with orbital ridges and nasal bridge felt anteriorly. Which ONE of the following is the most appropriate management?**

A. Caesarean section

B. Keillands forceps delivery

C. Mediolateral episiotomy

D. Rotational ventouse in the room

E. Trial of instrumental delivery in theatre

22. **A 15-year-old girl is admitted with abdominal pain. Last menstrual period was one week ago. She is requesting the morning-after pill. Which ONE of the following would you use to determine whether she is competent to receive contraception?**

A. Advanced directive

B. Fraser criteria

C. Gillick competence

D. Mental capacity act

E. Speak to her parents

23. **You are asked to review a 35-year-old woman's blood pressure on labour ward. She has just had a normal vaginal delivery and has lost approximately 300 ml blood only. You note she is rhesus negative. Which ONE of the following is the correct next step?**
    A. Administer 250 iu anti-D immunoglobulin as soon as possible
    B. Administer 250 iu anti-D immunoglobulin within 48 hours of delivery
    C. Administer 500 iu anti-D immunoglobulin within 72 hours of delivery
    D. Administer 500 iu anti-D immunoglobulin if the blood pressure is normal
    E. Perform a Kleihauer test

24. **A 36-year-old woman presents with acute onset chest pain. She is 32 weeks' pregnant in her first pregnancy. Her BMI is 34 and she has a known history of asthma. ECG suggests ST segment elevation myocardial infarction. Which ONE of the following is the most appropriate treatment for acute coronary syndrome?**
    A. Consider thrombolysis
    B. Deliver the baby then transfer to acute coronary unit
    C. Give aspirin 300 mg orally
    D. Give a GTN infusion (50 mg/ml)
    E. Perform a trial of vagal manoeuvres under continuous ECG

25. **A 29-year-old woman in her first pregnancy is admitted in labour at 4 cm, having broken her waters ten hours ago. A repeat vaginal examination shows she is 4 cm dilated four hours later, with contractions every 4–5 minutes. Which ONE of the following is the most appropriate next step for management?**
    A. Commence syntocinon
    B. Deliver by caesarean section
    C. Insert epidural
    D. Insert vaginal prostaglandin
    E. Repeat vaginal examination in 2 hours

26. **A 32-year-old woman is given syntocinon following a vaginal examination which showed she was persistently 8–9 cm with the head poorly applied to the cervix, despite having contractions every 3–4 minutes. This is her first pregnancy and she is 41 weeks gestation, undergoing an induction of labour for post-dates. Vaginal examination confirms she is 9 cm after syntocinon administration for 4 hours. She has an epidural in situ and foetal heart rate is 155 bpm. Which ONE of the following is the most appropriate next step for management?**
    A. Continue syntocinon for 2 hours
    B. Deliver by caesarean section within 30 minutes
    C. Deliver by caesarean section within 1 hour
    D. Increase syntocinon infusion rate for 2 hours
    E. Perform artificial rupture of membranes

27. You are called to see a 38-year-old woman in her second pregnancy at 39 weeks gestation. She has been pushing for almost two hours with epidural, contracting every three minutes. Abdominal examination confirms 0/5 palpable and CTG is normal. The position is occipito-anterial and the presenting part is at the ischial spines. Which **ONE** of the following is the most appropriate next step for management?

    A. Perform a caesarean section in the next hour
    B. Perform a caesarean-section in the next hour
    C. Perform a trial of instrumental delivery in theatre
    D. Perform a trial of instrumental delivery in the room
    E. Start syntocinon infusion

28. A 36-year-old woman is discharged home in her first pregnancy having been treated for severe **OHSS** in hospital, following **IVF**. Which **ONE** of the following risks are associated with pregnancy and **OHSS**?

    A. Caesarean section
    B. Intrauterine death
    C. Pre-eclampsia
    D. Placenta accreta
    E. Second trimester miscarriage

29. You are asked to discuss the delivery options with a 39-year-old woman in diabetic antenatal clinic whose growth ultrasound scan at 36 weeks gestation shows an estimated foetal weight of 4,100 g. In this case, when obtaining consent, which **ONE** of the following must doctors follow?

    A. Bolam test
    B. Fraser guidelines
    C. Gillick competence
    D. Montgomery ruling
    E. Sidaway test

30. A 29-year-old woman is admitted at 35 + 5 weeks gestation with confirmed prelabour rupture of membranes. She is medically fit and well and CTG is normal. This is her first pregnancy and upon reviewing her antenatal notes you see that she had a positive group **B** streptococcus test at 28 weeks gestation. What is the most appropriate plan of management?

    A. Caesarean section at 37 weeks gestation
    B. Cervical sweep and induction of labour in 48 hours
    C. Expectant management until 37 weeks gestation
    D. Immediate induction of labour
    E. Syntocinon at 36 weeks gestation

31. You are asked to see a 33-year-old woman in the day assessment unit who is attending with mastitis. She is tearful and wants to stop breastfeeding. Which ONE of the following is correct regarding breastfeeding?

    A. There is a reduced risk of gestational diabetes
    B. The risk of postmenopausal ovarian cancer is reduced in women who breastfeed
    C. The risk of eczema is reduced in breastfed babies
    D. The risk of postpartum haemorrhage is higher in women who breastfeed
    E. The contraceptive benefits of lactational amenorrhoea in an exclusively breastfed infant is 90% at 6 months

32. A GP calls you for contraceptive advice for a 23-year-old woman who is weaning her 6-month baby. She is breastfeeding her baby once a day and has had unprotected sexual intercourse two days ago. Which ONE of the following is correct?

    A. Insertion of the copper intrauterine device is contraindicated up to 28 days after delivery
    B. Insertion of the copper intrauterine device is contraindicated up to 3 months after delivery
    C. No additional contraception is required as this woman is breastfeeding regularly
    D. Women can continue breastfeeding after they have taken oral emergency contraception
    E. Women should avoid breastfeeding, express and discard milk for 5 days after they have taken oral emergency contraception

33. A 35-year-old woman comes to see you for longer-term contraceptive advice. She is not keen on oral contraception, having conceived her third child whilst taking it. Which ONE of the following has the lowest risk of an unintended pregnancy within the first year of use with typical use and perfect use?

    A. Copper intrauterine device
    B. Female sterilization
    C. Progestogen-only injectable (DMPA)
    D. Progestogen-only implant
    E. Vasectomy

34. A 38-year-old year old women with a BMI of 40 underwent planned elective third caesarean section. Following birth of the baby, a 4 cm long defect was noted in the anterior wall of the bladder. This defect was repaired in two layers by the on-call consultant obstetrician.

    Which one of the following is the appropriate postoperative management plan for bladder?

    A. Drain bladder for one week and remove the catheter
    B. Drain bladder for two weeks and remove the catheter
    C. Drain bladder for two weeks and arrange intravenous pyelogram before its removal
    D. Drain bladder for two weeks and arrange intravesical methylene blue dye instillation test before removing the catheter
    E. Drain bladder for two weeks and arrange retrograde cystogram before removing the catheter

35. A 32-year-old woman attends a colposcopy clinic following a smear test which shows glandular changes. She has previously had a **LLETZ** treatment at the age of 28. Which **ONE** of the following is correct?

A. Adequately treated CIN has a recurrence rate of 10% at two years

B. Colposcopy alone is adequate for the diagnosis of glandular lesions

C. Sampling of the transformation zone may be difficult after treatment

D. Smoking triples the risk of cervical cancer

E. Women should have annual smear tests for 5 years following a LLETZ treatment

36. A 25-year-old nulliparous woman is known to be **HIV** positive for 2 years has had a smear test showing high-risk **HPV**. Which **ONE** of the following is the most appropriate management?

A. Optimize HIV medications

B. Refer to colposcopy

C. Repeat the smear in 3 months

D. Repeat the smear in 6 months

E. Repeat the smear in 1 year

37. A 56-year-old woman attends clinic having had a hysterectomy and completely excised **CIN**. Which **ONE** of the following is correct?

A. She does not require any further smears

B. She should have a vaginal vault sample at 6 months; if this is HPV negative, she can be discharged

C. She should have a vaginal vault sample at 12 months; if this is HPV negative, she can be discharged

D. She should have a colposcopy in 6 months; if her smear is HPV negative, she can be discharged

E. She should have a colposcopy in 1 year; if her smear is HPV negative, she can be discharged

38. A 28-year-old woman presents with the results of her smear test. She is known to have an irregular menstrual cycle due to polycystic ovarian syndrome. She is taking the contraceptive pill to regulate her periods and has recently started a new sexual relationship. She smokes socially only. The cervical smear report states the following:

High-risk HPV infection, no dyskaryosis

Which **ONE** of the following is the most appropriate next step in managing this result?

A. HPV vaccination

B. Perform STI infection screen

C. Perform colposcopy

D. Repeat cervical smear in 3 years

E. Repeat cervical smear and HPV screening in one year

39. **A 26-year-old woman presents with the results of her first smear test. She is known to have herpes and has had a caesarean section for her first pregnancy six months ago. She is otherwise medically fit and well, with a regular menstrual cycle. She is not taking any contraception and has recently stopped breastfeeding. She smokes socially only. The cervical smear report states the following:**

    Mild dyskaryosis with high-risk HPV infection

    Which ONE of the following is the most appropriate next step in managing this result?

    A. HPV vaccination

    B. Prescribe the combined contraceptive pill

    C. Perform colposcopy

    D. Repeat cervical smear in 3 years

    E. Repeat cervical smear and HPV screening in 6 months

40. **A 52-year-old woman recently had a smear with her GP which has come back with the following result:**

    Inadequate cells for analysis

    She previously had a smear eight months ago with the same result and has previously had a LLETZ at the age of 32. She has regular periods with no changes to her vaginal discharge. What is the ONE most appropriate next course of action?

    A. Perform a vaginal infection screen to exclude infection

    B. Prescribe a course of oestrogen cream

    C. Prescribe a course of antibiotics

    D. Refer to colposcopy

    E. Repeat smear test in 3 months

41. **Which one of the following conditions does not cause electrolyte imbalance during first trimester of pregnancy?**

    A. Hyperemesis gravidarum

    B. Hyperthyroidism

    C. Dehydration

    D. Gestational diabetes

    E. Chronic renal failure

42. **Which one is the most important factor affecting acid-base balance during normal pregnancy?**

    A. Increased blood volume

    B. Increase renal blood flow

    C. Decreased plasma bicarbonate levels

    D. Increased respiratory rate

    E. Hormonal changes

43. A 35-year-old woman, who works at a farm, presents at 20 weeks of gestation with a diagnosis of primary CMV infection. She has requested an amniocentesis.

Which one of the following describes proportion of symptomatic babies at birth, while exposed to CMV infection *in utero*?

A. 10–15%
B. 10–25%
C. 25–35%
D. 35–45%
E. >45%

44. A 34-year-old woman who has had a baby 10 days ago would like to restart her combined pill for contraception. She is not breastfeeding but is taking antibiotics for endometritis following a manual removal of placenta. Which ONE of the following is correct?

A. She can commence the combined contraceptive pill immediately
B. She can commence the combined contraceptive pill at 3 weeks if she has risk factors for thrombosis
C. She can commence the combined contraceptive pill at 6 weeks if she has risk factors for thrombosis
D. She should consider insertion of the Mirena coil
E. She should consider insertion of the intrauterine device

45. A 39-year-old woman attends in her third pregnancy at 19 weeks of gestation. She has been informed that foetus has a Down syndrome. She is already looking after a child with developmental issues and feels she would be unable to cope with another child. She is requesting termination of pregnancy.

Which one of the following statutory grounds of Abortion Act applies in her case?

A. Statutory ground A
B. Statutory ground B
C. Statutory ground C
D. Statutory ground D
E. Statutory ground E

46. **A 38-year-old woman with a BMI of 40 is admitted in labour and wishes to speak with the anaesthetist to discuss various options for pain relief. Her sister suffered from severe headache following her recent delivery. She believes it was due to her epidural in labour.**

    Which one of the following figures represents the risk of a dural tap following an epidural block?

    A. 0.5%

    B. 0.5–1.5%

    C. 0.5–2.5%

    D. 2–4%

    E. 3–5%

47. **A 29-year-old woman with a BMI of 22 is admitted to the early assessment unit with a diagnosis of ruptured ectopic pregnancy. Her abdomen is distended. Her temperature is 36.4, pulse rate is 120 beats per minute, blood pressure 88/58 mmHg and less than 20 ml of dark urine in the bladder catheter bag. Her National Early Warning Score (NEWS) is 6.**

    Which one of the following should be used immediately while waiting for blood transfusion?

    A. 10% glucose

    B. Glucose 5% and furosemide 20 mg

    C. Sodium chloride 0.9%/5% glucose

    D. Sodium chloride 0.45%/4% glucose

    E. Sodium chloride 0.9%

48. **A 35-year-old woman with three previous caesarean sections is seen at 36 weeks gestation to arrange a planned elective caesarean section for placenta praevia grade 3 anterior. She refuses transfusion of blood and related products. She has signed a form so all healthcare professionals are aware of her religious beliefs and wishes.**

    Which one of the following applies to her?

    A. Living will

    B. Advance refusal

    C. Advance decision

    D. Consult the court

    E. Advance directive

49. **A 14-year-old schoolgirl with fully developed secondary sexual characteristics attends her general practitioner with history of irregular periods. She had unprotected intercourse with a school friend and her pregnancy test is positive. Her ultrasound scan confirms an 8 weeks gestation. She is requesting termination of pregnancy. She understands the risks involved in this process.**

    Which one of the following is the most important part of consultation?

    A. Inform social services

    B. Inform police

    C. Speak to the relevant authorities in the school

    D. Assess her Gillick competence

    E. Contact parents for their consent to proceed with her request

50. **A 18-year-old woman has been seen at the emergency department in considerable distress as she volunteers history of assault. A tear of vulva has been noted.**

    She has requested a forensic examination.

    Which one of the following is the most appropriate?

    A. Offer first aid and suture the tear of vulva

    B. Clean the affected area and then DNA samples can be taken

    C. Not to clean until DNA samples have been taken

    D. Take photographs and then clean and dress her

    E. Allow her to use a sanitary towel and pass urine if she wishes.

Extended Matching Questions

Options for Questions 1–5

For each case described, choose the single most likely answer from the list of options. Each option may be used once, more than once, or not at all.

Options:

  A. Feedback sandwich
  B. Kern's 6-step framework
  C. Miller's pyramid
  D. Mini-CEX
  E. Objective structured clinical examination
  F. Outcome 1
  G. Outcome 2
  H. Outcome 3
  I. Outcome 4
  K. Outcome 5
  L. Pendleton's model
  M. Short answer questions
  N. TO2

1. You are part of a team of obstetricians creating simulation training for perineal repair competencies for junior trainees. You are trying to create assessments that will examine their ability to define perineal tears at birth. Which model is used to depict attainment of mastery of skills, used when assessments are tailored to examine each of the levels?

2. When deciding which assessments can be used to assess repair competencies, you decide that a simulated assessment with a model would be the ideal method. What is a common method of assessing clinical competence in medical education?

3. When creating the plan for your training course, you find it difficult to think of specific learning outcomes, teaching content, and appropriate assessments. Which is a widely used method to develop medical education curricula across specialties?

4. Sheila, an ST5 trainee, has just received her ARCP outcome. It has outlined that she needs development of early pregnancy scanning, but that additional training time is not required. Her Postgraduate Dean (PGD) will ensure that her next attachment will be appropriate to achieve the necessary training opportunities. Sheila's CCT date is not altered.

5. Ram is a ST4 doctor, who performs an early pregnancy scan under direct observation. His trainer then puts aside time to provide feedback. She asks Ram what went well, and then tells Ram what she observed went well. She then probes Ram on what could be improved, with feedback on what she felt Ram could improve on. Which feedback model is the trainer's approach based on?

Options for Questions 6–10

For each case described next, choose the single most likely answer from the list of options. Each option may be used once, more than once, or not at all.

Options:

  A. Anterior pituitary gland
  B. Broad ligament

C. Cardinal ligaments

D. Inferior 1/3 of the rectum

E. Inferior 1/3 of the rectum and anus

F. Inferior 2/3 of the rectum

G. L1

H. L2

I. L3

J. L4

K. Posterior pituitary gland

L. Round ligaments

M. Suspensory ligament

N. Utero-ovarian ligament

6. A 23-year-old nulliparous lady is in labour at 40 weeks gestation, having broken her waters 6 hours ago. Her contractions have slowed down to 1 in 10 minutes. You discuss the possibility of starting syntocinon to help with her contractions. She asks you what syntocinon is. Where is oxytocin released from?

7. You are asked to organize an urgent laparoscopic ovarian cystectomy for a 26-year-old woman with suspected ovarian torsion. At which position does the ovarian artery originate from on the abdominal aorta?

8. You are asked to review a 29-year-old woman who has sustained a third-degree tear during a normal vaginal delivery and is bleeding heavily. Which of the following does the middle rectal artery supply?

9. A 45-year-old patient pre-diabetic patient attends her GP with recurrent abscesses of the labia majora. She has previously had incision and drainage of collections twice. She is given a course of antibiotics. Which ligament passes through the inguinal canal and inserts into the labia majora?

10. You are in theatre assisting the subspeciality trainee perform a vaginal hysterectomy. Which of the following is the first ligament to be clamped in a vaginal hysterectomy?

Options for Questions 11–15

For each case described below, choose the single most likely cause from the list of options. Each option may be used once, more than once, or not at all.

Options:

A. Amniotic fluid embolism

B. Cardiomyopathy

C. Chest infection

D. Diabetic ketoacidosis

E. Haemorrhage

F. HELLP syndrome

G. Myocardial infarction

H. Placental abruption

I. Pneumonia

J. Pulmonary embolus

K. Pulmonary hypertension

L. Sepsis

M. Substance misuse

N. Suicide

11. A healthy 27-year-old woman presents at 36 weeks gestation in her first pregnancy with shortness of breath and worsening chest pain. Her brother died unexpectedly aged 19 years. Chest X-ray shows an enlarged heart. When you see her, she is sweating with cool peripheries. Bi-basal pulmonary crackles are present on chest auscultation, with a raised JVP. Oxygen saturation is 84% on air and her heart rate is 115 bpm.

12. You are called to see a 25-year-old woman in recovery who complains of numbness and tingling after an emergency caesarean section for foetal distress following an induction of labour. Estimated blood loss was 1.2 L. As you arrive, she collapses following a seizure. She is medically fit and well with no history of epilepsy. Blood pressure is 70/40.

13. A 24-year-old woman presents to accident and emergency feeling generally unwell, with blurred vision. She has vomited three times since admission and feels lethargic. She is an insulin dependent diabetic, currently 26 weeks gestation in her first pregnancy. When you approach her, she is hyperventilating, unable to give a coherent history and you note her breath smells like pear drops. Blood pressure is 68/45 and heart rate is 112 bpm.

14. A 25-year-old woman presents with a rash, dry cough, and worsening shortness of breath in accident and emergency. She is 34 weeks gestation in her second pregnancy. Her son has just contracted chicken pox at school. She is experiencing pain on inhalation. Examination confirms a temperature of 38°C and coarse crackles on auscultation.

15. A 28-year-old woman presents at 29 weeks gestation after a fall. This is her first pregnancy and she is medically fit and well. She is pale and sweaty, complaining of severe constant lower abdominal pain. Abdominal examination confirms a uterus which feels hard and tender to touch. CTG shows a foetal heart rate of 100 bpm.

Options for Questions 16–20

For each case described next, choose the single most likely cause from the list of options. Each option may be used once, more than once, or not at all.

Options:

    A. Bladder injury

    B. Damage to bowel

    C. Failure to gain entry into abdominal cavity

    D. Failure to identify disease

    E. Failure to visualize uterine cavity

    F. Faecal or flatus incontinence

    G. Haemorrhage requiring blood transfusion

    H. Haemorrhage requiring return to theatre

    I. Intrauterine adhesions

    J. Premature menopause

    K. Removal of ovaries

    L. Urinary incontinence

    M. Uterine perforation

    N. Ureteric injury

16. A 56-year-old woman is listed for diagnostic hysteroscopy following a postmenopausal bleed. She has had two caesarean sections, a transcervical resection of fibroids and a previous uterine ablation for menorrhagia. She is diabetic and her BMI is 40.

17. A 32-year-old woman has an instrumental delivery of a baby weighing 4105 g. A grade 3C tear of the anal sphincter is identified and repaired using 3/0 PDS.

18. A 46-year-old multiparous woman is scheduled for abdominal hysterectomy because of menorrhagia and urinary frequency. Her uterus is enlarged equivalent to 28 weeks gestation.

19. You are consenting a 19-year-old woman for her second surgical management of miscarriage.

20. A 36-year-old woman presents in her first pregnancy at 36 weeks gestation. She has come to antenatal clinic to discuss the risks of a planned caesarean and vaginal birth. Which ONE risk is halved by having a planned caesarean section rather than a vaginal birth?

Options for Questions 21–25

For each of the following clinical scenarios, choose the most appropriate management option from the list provided. Each option may be used once, more than once, or not at all.

Options:

A. Bladder scan
B. Chest X-ray
C. CT abdomen and pelvis
D. CT angio abdomen
E. CT urogram
F. Cystogram
G. Intermittent self-catheterization
H. Intravenous pyelogram
I. MRI pelvis
J. Plain X-ray abdomen
K. Transvaginal ultrasound scan
L. Urea and electrolytes
M. Urinary catecholamines
N. Urinary catheterization

21. A 70-year-old had hysteroscopy for postmenopausal bleeding. She had drainage of pyometra and removal of a large endometrial polyp. She has been readmitted 48 hours later with temperature of 39°C and an acute abdomen.

22. A 38-year-old woman had a laparoscopic hysterectomy and left salpingo-oophorectomy for ovarian endometrioma. It was a technically challenging operation. Postoperative recovery was uneventful but she was readmitted 96 hours later feeling unwell and complaining of pain in left loin and constipation.

23. A 50-year-old woman had a total abdominal hysterectomy and bilateral salpingo-oophorectomy for a large uterine fibroid of 16 weeks size. She was seen for postoperative follow-up six weeks later. She is complaining of excessive discharge per vagina.

24. A 72-year-old woman had surgery for grade 3 vaginal prolapse comprising of a vaginal hysterectomy, anterior and posterior repair with Sacrospinous fixation. Total operating time was 150 minutes with blood loss of 450 grams. When reviewed 12 hours later, there was 30 ml urine in the bag.

25. A 55-year-old had a transvaginal tape procedure. 12 hours later she was unable to pass urine following removal of indwelling catheter.

Options for Questions 26–30

For each of the following clinical scenarios, choose the most appropriate management option from the list provided. Each option may be used once, more than once, or not at all.

Options:

    A. Change to heparinoid danaparoid sodium

    B. Change to low molecular heparin (LMWH)

    C. Change to prophylactic intravenous unfractionated heparin

    D. Close surveillance antenatally and prophylactic LMWH postnatally for 6 weeks

    E. Commence dalteparin

    F. Commence prophylactic LMWH

    G. Low-dose aspirin antenatally

    H. Monitor anti-Xa levels

    I. No treatment

    J. Prophylactic LMWH antenatally and postnatally for 14 days

    K. Prophylactic LMWH antenatally and postnatally for 6 weeks

    L. TED stockings

    M. Therapeutic dose of LMWH antenatally

    N. Therapeutic dose of LMWH antenatally and postnatally

26. A 30-year-old woman with a BMI of 25 attends antenatal clinic at 12 weeks of gestation. Her booking bloods are normal. She has a known history of varicose veins.

27. A 28-year-old woman with a BMI of 22 attends her antenatal booking visit at 12 weeks gestation. She volunteers a past history of unprovoked venous thromboembolism four years ago. Her thrombophilia screening is negative. There is no relevant family history.

28. A 30-year-old woman with a BMI of 34 attends antenatal clinic at 28 weeks gestation for review. She was diagnosed with left-sided DVT at 18 weeks of gestation and she is currently on LMWH. Her blood count shows haemoglobin of 140 gm/dl and a platelet count of 68 × 109/dl.

29. A 38-year-old woman with a BMI of 35 attends the antenatal clinic at 12 weeks gestation. Her ultrasound scan confirms an intrauterine singleton pregnancy. She volunteers a history of a single episode of left brachial artery thrombosis four years ago while she was travelling back from Australia. No cause was found following thorough investigations.

30. A 35-year-old woman with a BMI of 22 attends for her booking visit in her second pregnancy at 15 weeks gestation. During her first pregnancy, she developed pre-eclampsia. Her baby weighed 3.4 kg at birth. She gives a history of deep venous thrombosis 18 months ago following a long holiday flight and was treated with warfarin for six months. She has been prescribed low-dose aspirin by the district midwife.

Options for Questions 31–35

For each of the following clinical scenarios, choose the most appropriate management option from the list provided. Each option may be used once, more than once, or not at all.

Options:

    A. Bladder injury

    B. Bowel injury

    C. Bradycardia

    D. Inferior epigastric vessel injury

    E. Injury to external iliac vessel

    F. Injury to internal iliac vessel

    G. Intraoperative pain

    H. Omental injury

I.   Postoperative pain

J.   Pulmonary embolism

K.   Tachycardia

L.   Ureteric injury

M.   Uterine perforation

N.   Vasovagal shock

31. A 35-year-old woman with a BMI of 30 who had three previous caesarean sections is being investigated for chronic pelvic pain. Her CT scan is suggestive of adhesions. She was admitted for operative laparoscopy for possible adhesiolysis. The trocar was introduced via Hassan's technique. Laparoscopy showed yellow frothy fluid in the abdominal cavity.

32. A 42-year-old woman with a BMI of 20 was diagnosed with a right ovarian cyst of 7 cm diameter. She has requested laparoscopic removal of this cyst. Verres needle was inserted via infra-umbilical route to create a pneumoperitoneum. Once the laparoscope was introduced, the anaesthetist noted that her blood pressure dropped to 100/58 mmHg and her pulse was 100 beats per minutes. Her bowel appeared to be a rather dusky blue.

33. A 35-year-old woman with a BMI of 32 has been admitted for laparoscopic sterilization. Once the second port was inserted laterally, brisk bleeding was noted in the abdomen.

34. A 38-year-old woman with BMI of 24 had operative laparoscopy for stage 3 pelvic endometriosis, requiring extensive adhesiolysis in the pelvis and left lateral pelvic wall followed by removal of left ovarian endometrioma. She was readmitted seven days later with tachycardia, and moderate abdominal distension. Her blood urea is significantly elevated and ultrasound scan has shown free fluid in the abdomen.

35. A 45-year-old woman underwent a diagnostic hysteroscopy and resection of a sub-mucus fibroid measuring 4 cm in diameter. The operating procedure was described as challenging. Six hours later, her pulse was 100 beats per minute and she is complaining of abdominal and pelvic pains which is unresponsive to oral analgesia. She is also experiencing moderate vaginal bleeding. An ultrasound scan showed free fluid in the pelvis measuring about 150 ml.

Options for Questions 36–40

For each of the following clinical scenarios, choose the most appropriate management option from the list provided. Each option may be used once, more than once, or not at all.

Options:

A.   Canesten vaginally

B.   Canesten vaginally and oral itraconazole

C.   Cephalosporin

D.   Doxycycline

E.   Erythromycin

F.   Flucloxacillin

G.   Fluconazole

H.   Metronidazole

I.   Ofloxacin and Metronidazole

J.   Penicillin

K.   Penicillin and Metronidazole

L.   Penicillin and probiotics vaginally

M.   Piperacillin

N.   Teicoplanin

36. An 18-year-old woman presents with history of episodes of recurrent vaginal discharge for the past 12 months treated with various drugs. Vaginal discharge shows inflamed vulva with profuse vaginal discharge with diffuse fishy smell. A high vaginal swab grows profuse growth of Group B Streptococcus Agalactiae (GBS) and Gardnerella vaginalis.

37. A 20-year-old nulliparous woman, presents with history of recurrent non-smelly vaginal discharge. She is experiencing burning sensation and superficial dyspareunia for the past 12 months. She has been self-treating with oral fluconazole with temporary relief of symptoms. Examination shows non-offensive cottage cheese like discharge. Her STI screening test is negative. Inspection of the vulva shows erythema, fissuring, and local oedema.

38. A 22-year-old woman presents at the gynaecology department with a right sided swelling in the lower part of the vagina. She tells you that it has increased slightly in size following intercourse 24 hours ago. There is no vaginal discharge and her temperature is 37°C.

39. A 24-year-old woman presents with lower abdominal pain and vaginal discharge. She is feeling unwell. On examination, her vaginal discharge is grey/green coloured coating the vaginal wall with no redness. Her bimanual examination demonstrates tenderness in both adnexae.

40. A 28-year-old woman has just returned from holiday and is now presenting with a history of dysuria, intense pain following voiding urine, mucopurulent vaginal discharge, and postcoital spotting. Speculum examination shows endocervical ulcers and contact bleeding from the cervix.

Options for Questions 41–45

For each of the following clinical scenarios, choose the most appropriate management option from the list provided. Each option may be used once, more than once, or not at all.

Options:

 A. Consent by the patient
 B. Consent by the partner
 C. Consent from the court required
 D. Decline post-mortem
 E. Human Rights Act
 F. No consent required
 G. No registration of stillbirth required
 H. Not to proceed with the surgery
 I. Post-mortem is required by law
 J. Post-mortem recommended
 K. Register as neonatal death
 L. Register as stillbirth
 M. Registered under the Abortion Act 1967
 N. Wishes of mother/parents needs to be respected

41. A 13-year-old young girl has been brought to the accident and emergency department with acute pain over the last 24 hours, worsened by her period. A clinical and radiological assessment confirms acute appendicitis. Consultant surgeon has recommended immediate surgery.

42. A 16-year-old woman is admitted to labour ward with strong uterine contractions. This is a concealed and unbooked pregnancy. She is accompanied with a female friend. Clinical

examination suggests that uterine size is consistent with 30 weeks gestation. An ultrasound scan shows a singleton live baby. She delivers four hours later, and the baby requires admission to the neonatal unit, where she passes away 24 hours later. A post-mortem examination has been recommended. This investigation is not allowed in her religion.

43. A 42-year-old woman had assisted conception treatment and at 18 weeks gestation undergoes selective foeticide for an abnormal baby. She is admitted with a diagnosis of placental abruption at 30 weeks and is delivered by emergency caesarean section; one live healthy premature baby and a tiny dead foetus.

44. A 19-year-old woman presents at the labour ward at 23 weeks of gestation with strong uterine contraction and preterm premature rupture of membranes. She delivers a live baby weighing 400 grams. The baby dies 24 hours later in the neonatal unit.

45. A 28-year-old woman undergoes emergency caesarean section under general anaesthesia at maternal request. Following completion of the caesarean section, a previously unknown left ovarian cyst of 5–6 cm in diameter is noted which appears to be a dermoid cyst.

Options for Questions 46–50

For each of the following clinical scenarios, choose the correct injury option from the list provided. Each option may be used once, more than once, or not at all.

Options:

A. Common perineal nerve

B. Femoral nerve

C. Genitofemoral nerve

D. Iliohypogastric nerve

E. Ilio-inguinal nerve

F. Inferior rectal nerve

G. Lateral cutaneous nerve

H. Obturator nerve

I. Pelvic splachic nerves

J. Pudendal nerve

K. Sacral splanchic nerve

L. Sciatic nerve

M. Superior rectal nerve

N. Tibial nerve

46. A 48-year-old woman, with a BMI of 45, underwent major abdomino-pelvic debulking surgery for stage 3 ovarian cancer involving anterior resection. She is complaining of weakness of her hip movements. On examination, there is paraesthesia over the anterior and medial aspect of right thigh.

47. A 45-year-old non-white woman with a BMI of 44 who had three previous caesarean sections, undergoes hysterectomy for a 14-weeks sized uterus studded with multiple fibroids. It was a technically challenging operation and required extension of lower transverse incision laterally. She is now complaining of sharp burning pain to the left labia and thigh.

48. A 44-year-old woman with a BMI of 30 had a Wertheim hysterectomy carried out for cervical cancer stage 1B. She now presents with a history of burning sensation and sometimes shooting or throbbing pain in the labia majora and mons pubis. Sometimes pelvic pain is also felt in the lower back and between legs.

49. A 25-year-old, 30 weeks pregnant woman with a BMI of 28 presents at the emergency obstetric clinic complaining of sudden onset of mild ache in her lower back, which travels through the hips and buttocks in the right leg. Sometimes it feels like an electric shock. She is also complaining of tingling in the right leg. There is no history of trauma or accident.

50. A 28-year-old Para 1 is in second stage of labour and her vaginal examination confirms that the vertex is in occipito-anterior position and 2 cm below the ischial spine. The on-call consultant decides to use a local pelvic block to deliver the baby by ventouse in the room.

Single Best Answers

1. A. Coagulation

Coagulation uses a pulsed waveform with a high voltage. The waveform is at a lower average power, not generating enough heat for explosive vaporization, but enough for thermal coagulation. The sparks spread over a wide area causes charring rather than cutting.

Balog J, et al. Intraoperative tissue identification using rapid evaporative ionization mass spectrometry. *Sci Transl Med* 2013;5(194):194ra93.

2. C. Left colic artery

Left colic artery is a branch of the inferior mesenteric artery. The jejunal, ileocolic, and right colic arteries are branches of the superior mesenteric arteries. The ovarian artery is a lateral visceral branch of the abdominal aorta.

3. D. Death from age 7 days to 27 completed days of life

Early neonatal death is death in the first 6 days of life. Late neonatal death is death from age 7 days to 27 completed days of life.

RCOG Green-top guideline 55: Late intrauterine fetal death and stillbirth; 2010.

4. A. Adenine

The purine amino acid DNA bases are adenine and guanine, while the pyramidine DNA bases are cytosine and thymine.

5. D. 60 to 99 degrees Celsius

Radiofrequencies are generated by diathermy heat tissues, by creating intracellular oscillation. At 60 degrees cell death or fulguration occurs, at 60 to 99 degrees dehydration of tissue cells occur along with coagulation, and at around 100 degrees, vaporization or cutting occurs.

6. C. Deep transverse perineal muscles

The contents of the deep perineal pouch include the external urethral sphincter muscles, deep transverse perineal muscles, internal pudendal vessel, and dorsal nerve of the clitoris. The superficial perineal pouch includes the root (crura) of the clitoris and ischiocaverbosus, bulbs of the vestibules, bulbospongiosus, greater vestibular glands, superficial transverse perineal muscles, branches of internal pudendal vessels and perineal nerves all form the contents of the superficial perineal pouch.

7. E. Pulsed waveform with high voltage

Cutting uses continuous waveform with a low voltage. Coagulation alternatively uses pulsed waveforms with high voltage.

Balog J, et al. Intraoperative tissue identification using rapid evaporative ionization mass spectrometry. *Sci Transl Med* 2013;5(194):194ra93.

8. B. 1–14%

There is a risk of chronic post-vasectomy pain (CPVP), a postoperative testicular, scrotal, penile, or lower abdominal pain that occurs more than 3 months after the procedure and is rarely severe and persistent in some men. The incidence rate of CPVP ranges from 1 to 14%.

FSRH. Male and female sterilisation: summary of recommendations. Faculty of Sexual and Reproductive Healthcare; 2014.

9. B. 2.4–7.3 per 1,000 procedures

The risk varies depending on the method used, but the 10-year cumulative probability of ectopic pregnancy ranges from 2.4 to 7.3 per 1,000 procedures.

FSRH. Male and female sterilisation: summary of recommendations. Faculty of Sexual and Reproductive Healthcare; 2014.

10. C. Speak to the midwife co-ordinator about the situation and call your consultant.

The baby you are managing needs delivery regardless of whether the patient stops pushing. The confounding risks in this scenario is that doing a trial may then end up in a c-section, while there are two other patients on oxytocin which may be complicated by foetal distress. Speaking to the midwife co-ordinator will make her aware that while waiting for the consultant on-call, she can manage the labourers on oxytocin, stopping oxytocin if necessary. You may need your consultant to be present in case of a haemorrhage with your trial, or if a caesarean section is required. Having insight and preparing your consultant for the potential outcomes, elicits good teamwork and communication.

NICE Guideline 190: Intrapartum care for healthy women and babies; 2014, updated 2022.

11. B. The risk to patient safety if working while tired.

As a doctor, the care of the patient is your main concern, and therefore your own health has to be looked after in order to provide good patient care. Whilst the other options are probably considerations when reporting, a poor reference should not be one. Each trust has a guardian of safe working who can provide further information of exception reporting.

12. D. Levator ani

The perineal body is a point of attachment for muscle fibres from the pelvic floor and the perineum itself: levator ani, bulbospongiosus muscle, superficial and deep transverse perineal muscles, external anal sphincter muscle, and external urethral sphincter muscle fibres.

13. D. Defect in 17α-hydroxylase

Deficiency in 21α-hydroxylase accounts for approximately 90% of CAH cases. Deficiencies in 11β-hydroxylase accounts for 5–8% and 17α-hydroxylase defects are rare. CAH is one of the most common autosomal recessive metabolic diseases.

Ahmed M, Bashir M, Okunoye GO, Konje JC. Adrenal disease and pregnancy: an overview. *TOG* 2021;23:265–77.

14. E. Thiamine

Thiamine (vitamin B1) deficiency causes Beriberi disease. Wet beriberi affects the cardiovascular system, while dry beriberi affects the central nervous system. Treatment includes re-introduction of thiamine via diet and supplements.

Felson S. What is beriberi? 2023. Available at: https://www.webmd.com/brain/what-is-beriberi

15. B. Acute early

Host versus graft rejection response is divided into acute early, which occurs in less than 10 days, acute late, which occurs after 10 days, and chronic which occurs after years of the transplant procedure due to failure of immunosuppression.

BMJ (2023). Graft-versus-host disease—symptoms, diagnosis and treatment. BMJ Best Practice; 2023. Available at: https://bestpractice.bmj.com/topics/en-gb/946

16. B. After ABC, call for help while assessing if the bleeding is caused by trauma, tissue, tone, or thrombus (4Ts)

As it states that the bleeding is ongoing and you are still in the room, you need to call for help from your midwifery colleagues and doctors. While she may not need to go to theatre yet, you need help to do basic observations, and help to administer drugs to help with bleeding depending on which of the '4Ts' you think is the cause. Starting with the basic ABC and determining the cause of bleeding is important. You may also need another intravenous line to start medication. You will also need help to massage the uterus and help with tone if atony is contributing. If, despite intervention, she continues to bleed, then a decision can be made to transfer the patient to theatre.

RCOG Green-top Guideline No. 52. Prevention and management of postpartum haemorrhage; 2016.

17. A. Situation, background, assessment, recommendation

SBAR is a communication tool or technique used by healthcare professionals to share patients' information effectively, especially during critical changes in a patient's status. It was developed by the US military for nuclear submarines where concise and relevant information was essential for safety. This easy to remember acronym frames conversations, when requiring a clinician's immediate attention and action.

NHS England. SBAR Communication Tool—Online Library of Quality, Service Improvement and Redesign Tools situation, background, assessment, Recommendation NHS England and NHS Improvement, p. 3; 2021. Available at: https://www.england.nhs.uk/wp-content/uploads/2021/03/qsir-sbar-communication-tool.pdf

18. B. Inadequate progress—additional training time required

Outcome 3 means that the trainee shows inadequate progress and therefore additional training time is given for ST5.

RCOG. Advice on ARCP outcomes; 2020. Available at: https://rcog.org.uk/careers-and-training/start ing-your-og-career/specialty-training/assessment-and-progression-through-training/arcp-annual-review-of-competence-progression/advice-on-arcp-outcomes/

19. C. DOPS

Direct observation of physical skill (DOPS) assessments are best suited to assess a trainee's technical, operational, or professional skills. Within obstetrics and gynaecology, the assessment method used for technical skills is called OSATS (objective structured assessment of technical skills), a tool very similar to DOPS which is used in other specialities.

RCOG. Workplace-based assessments (WPBAs) (n.d.). Available at: https://www.rcog.org.uk/careers-and-training/starting-your-og-career/specialty-training/assessment-and-progression-through-training/workplace-based-assessments-wpbas/

20. A. Internalized racism

Systemic/institutional racism, is differential access to 'capital' (e.g. housing, education, healthcare, employment, etc.) because Black and Brown bodies, minds, and cultures are perceived as less worthy. This explains an uneven playing field.

Interpersonal racism, and direct discrimination, is where one individual is racist towards another. This form of discrimination may be explicit or implicit; for example, race-based hate crimes and microaggression based on race.

Internalized level, explains how individuals from minority backgrounds accept the dominant, damaging racist narratives about their abilities and worth. They may disassociate from their own culture to survive. This leads to inferiority and resignation.

Okolo ID, et al. A race to the finish line. *Obstet Gynecol* 2023;25:92–96.

21. **A.** Caesarean section

Brow presentation is a form of cephalic presentation in which the head is midway between flexion and extension. It occurs in approximately 1 in 1,000 cases of labour. Vaginal examination can reveal frontal bones, supraorbital ridges, and the root of the nose but not the chin and the engagement diameter is mentovertical (13.5 cm). This is longer than the diameter of the pelvic inlet so a caesarean section is indicated. Whilst brow presentation may be transient, here abdominal examination confirmed 1/5 palpable, so a trial of instrumental delivery is contraindicated.

RCOG. *Basic practical skills in obstetrics and gynaecology.* Cambridge: Cambridge University Press; 2017.

22. **B.** Fraser criteria

Gillick competence is used to identify patients under the age of 16 who are capable of giving consent to any treatment. Fraser guidelines give the criteria to be met in order to give contraceptive advice or treatment without parental consent. The key principles for valid consent are competence, sufficient information to make a choice, and consent must be given voluntarily.

FSRH. Service standards on obtaining valid consent in SRH services; 2018.

RCOG. Management, governance and training online: Consent.

23. **C.** Administer 500 iu anti-D immunoglobulin within 72 hours of delivery

Delivery of any mode is a potentially sensitizing event in pregnancy. Routine postpartum administration of anti-D immunoglobulin within 72 hours of delivery significantly reduces the rate of alloimmunization. Further reduction in the sensitization rate can be achieved by routine antenatal prophylaxis in the third trimester of pregnancy.

British Committee for Standards in Haematology, Guideline on anti-D administration in pregnancy; 2014.

24. **C.** Give aspirin 300 mg orally

Acute coronary syndrome (ACS) comprises unstable angina, non-ST segment elevation, and ST segment elevation myocardial infarction. 300 mg aspirin should be given orally and is not contraindicated in pregnancy. GTN may be administered sublingually, but not as an infusion, which may cause hypotension. Whilst thrombolysis is not contraindicated and does not cross the placenta, it is not indicated for STEMI in pregnancy as the diagnosis may be aortic dissection. The immediate treatment of ACS should not be delayed for delivery. Ideally, delivery should be postponed if feasible for at least two weeks after an acute cardiac event. Vagal manoeuvres should be performed where the patient has been found to have a supraventricular tachycardia, not ACS.

Burns R, Dent K. *ALSG: Managing medical and obstetrics emergencies and trauma: a practical approach,* 4th ed. Oxford: Wiley-Blackwell; 2022

Nelson-Piercy C. *Obstetric medicine,* 6th ed. Boca Raton: CRC Press; 2020.

25. A. Commence syntocinon

Once delay in the established first stage is suspected, parity, cervical dilatation, and rate of change, uterine contractions, station and position of presenting part in conjunction with the woman's wishes need to be considered. All aspects of progress in labour should be assessed, including rate of cervical dilatation, descent, and rotation of the baby's head and the nature and frequency of contractions. Use of syntocinon after rupture of membranes will bring forward the time of birth but does not influence the mode of birth or other outcomes.

NICE Guideline 190. Intrapartum care for healthy women and babies; 2014; updated 2022.

26. C. Deliver by caesarean section within 1 hour

This is the most appropriate next step as she has been on syntocinon for four hours with regular contractions but no change to cervical findings. A cervical dilatation of less than 2 cm more after 4 hours of oxytocin warrants an obstetric review. Here, labour dystocia may be secondary to a malpresentation or a big baby. As the CTG is normal, delivery can occur within 1 hour (category 2, caesarean section). Artificial rupture of membranes should be performed prior to starting syntocinon.

NICE Guideline 190. Intrapartum care for healthy women and babies; 2014; updated 2022.

27. C. Perform a trial of instrumental delivery in theatre

For a multiparous woman, birth should take place within 2 hours of the start of the active second stage in most women. Oxytocin should be considered if contractions are inadequate at the onset of the second stage. Delivery should be in theatre given the presenting part is at the ischial spines. It is worth repeating the abdominal and vaginal examinations in theatre, as the presenting part and presentation may alter. Here, there is the possibility of instrumental delivery although this also depends on factors such as the CTG findings, maternal effort, and consent.

NICE Guideline 190. Intrapartum care for healthy women and babies; 2014; updated 2022.

28. C. Pre-eclampsia

Pregnancies complicated by OHSS may be at increased risk of pre-eclampsia and preterm delivery. Risks of pregnancy associated with IVF include multiple births, premature delivery, and low birth weight, ovarian hyperstimulation syndrome, ectopic pregnancy, miscarriage, and birth defects.

RCOG Green-top Guideline 5. The Management of ovarian hyperstimulation syndrome; 2016.

29. D. Montgomery ruling

When obtaining consent for treatment, the information given to a patient must be reasonable from the perspective of a reasonable person in the patient's position. This is the ruling following the Montgomery case, which replaces the tests founded in Bolam and refined in Sidaway. This includes assessing the effect of the patient's individual clinical circumstances on the probability of a benefit or harm occurring. Prior to Montgomery, a doctor's duty was to warn patients of risks based on whether they had acted in line with a responsible body of medical opinion.

GMC. Decision making and consent; 2020.

RCOG. Clinical governance 6: obtaining valid consent; 2015.

30. D. Immediate induction of labour

If a woman has preterm prelabour rupture of membranes after 34 + 0 weeks but before 37 weeks gestation and has a positive group B streptococcus test at any time in their current pregnancy, offer immediate induction of labour or caesarean birth.

NICE guideline 207. Inducing labour; 2021.

31. C. The risk of eczema is reduced in breastfed babies

The benefits of breastfeeding for the infant includes a reduction in gastrointestinal illness, respiratory infection, and acute otitis media. In the longer term, it can reduce atopic illnesses and allergies as well as type I diabetes. Benefits for the mother include a reduced risk of hypertension, type 2 diabetes, and premenopausal ovarian cancer. The contraceptive benefits of lactational amenorrhoea in a fully breastfed infant is nearly 99% effective at 6 months and 97% effective at 12 months, providing the mother is amenorrhoeic.

FRSH Guideline. Emergency contraception; 2012, amended 2020.

OGRM Barnes S, Bennett S, Datta S. Breastfeeding: debunking preconceptions and removing barriers; 2022.

32. A. Insertion of the copper intrauterine device is contraindicated up to 28 days after delivery

The contraceptive benefits of lactational amenorrhoea in a fully breast-fed infant is nearly 99% effective at 6 months and 97% effective at 12 months, providing the mother is amenorrhoeic. Contraception is required if full breastfeeding ceases, as in this case, or if menstruation returns. Breastfeeding women have a higher relative risk of uterine perforation during insertion of intrauterine contraception than non-breastfeeding women. However, the absolute risk of perforation is low and insertion of a copper intrauterine device is relatively contraindicated between 48 hours and 28 days after delivery due to the possible increased risk of uterine perforation and expulsion. Breastfeeding women should avoid breastfeeding, express and discard milk for a week after taking emergency oral contraception.

FRSH Guideline. Emergency contraception; 2012, amended 2020.

OGRM Barnes S, Bennett S, Datta S. Breastfeeding: debunking preconceptions and removing barriers; 2022.

33. D. Progestogen-only implant

The percentage of women experiencing an unintended pregnancy within the first year of use with typical and perfect use is as follows (FSRH UKMEC criteria, 2019): No method: Typical use 85%, perfect use 85%. Fertility awareness based methods: Typical use 24%, perfect use 0.4–5%. Progestogen only injectable, DMPA: Typical use 6%, perfect use 0.2%. Copper bearing intrauterine device: Typical use 0.8%, perfect use 0.6%. Levonorgestrel releasing intrauterine system: Typical use 0.2%, perfect use 0.2%. Progestogen only implant: Typical use 0.05%, perfect use 0.05%. Female sterilization: Typical use 0.5%, perfect use 0.5%. Vasectomy: Typical use 0.15%, perfect use: 0.1%. (Source: data from FSRH UKMEC criteria, 2016, amended 2019. Faculty of Sexual and Reproductive Healthcare 2006 to 2016.)

34. E. Drain bladder for two weeks and arrange retrograde cystogram before removing the catheter

Bladder should be freely drained for two weeks using a Foley's catheter. As the defect is quite significant, it is important to ensure that the defect has healed completely by organizing a retrograde cystogram. In this test, radio-opaque dye is injected to ensure that bladder walls are intact. If there is any doubt, Foley's catheter should be left for another week for free drainage and an opinion be sought from a consultant urologist as well.

Manidip P, Soma B. Cesarean bladder injury—obstetrician's nightmare. *J Family Med Prim Care* 2020;9(9):4526–4529.

35. C. Sampling of the transformation zone may be difficult after treatment

Adequately treated CIN has a recurrence rate of 5% at two years. Smoking doubles the risk of cervical cancer. Colposcopy alone lacks the sensitivity for the diagnosis of glandular lesions.

Public Health England. Updated cervical screening programme and colposcopy management guide; 2020.

36. B. Refer to colposcopy

Women with a new diagnosis of HIV and an abnormal cervical smear result should be regarded as high risk and reviewed in the colposcopy clinic.

Public Health England. Updated cervical screening programme and colposcopy management guide; 2020.

37. B. She should have a vaginal vault sample at 6 months; if this is HPV negative, she can be discharged

Women who have had a hysterectomy with CIN present may potentially develop vaginal intraepithelial neoplasia (VaIN) and invasive vaginal disease. For those with no CIN in their hysterectomy specimen and a normal smear history, no vaginal vault sample is required. For women who have had a hysterectomy and have completely excised CIN, a vaginal vault sample should be performed at 6 months following their hysterectomy—if the HPV result is negative, they can be discharged. Those who are high-risk HPV positive at 6 months should be referred to colposcopy. If CIN is incompletely excised, vault smears should be performed at 6 monthly intervals until 65 years of age or until 10 years after surgery.

Public Health England. Updated cervical screening programme and colposcopy management guide; 2020.

38. E. Repeat cervical smear and HPV screening in one year

Whilst vaccination can help prevent infection with certain strands of HPV (usually HPV 6, 11, 16, 18), it is not recommended whilst infection is present. A STI infection screen will not investigate or treat the abnormal smear findings. Colposcopy is not warranted at this stage because there is no dyskaryosis, simply HPV infection which may resolve spontaneously over time. Given the findings on smear show HPV infection only, the most appropriate management, in this case, is to repeat cervical smear and HPV screening in one year. Repeat cervical smear in 3 years is inappropriate given the findings of HPV infection, as this can affect the cells on the cervix over time.

Public Health England. Updated cervical screening programme and colposcopy management guide; 2020.

39. C. Perform colposcopy

Colposcopy is the most appropriate management plan. A colposcopy clinic is a specialist clinic which involves inspecting the cervix using a colposcope, applying solutions to inspect the severity of changes on the cervix, and considering whether to take a biopsy. This assessment directs whether further treatment is warranted. Whilst vaccination can help prevent infection with certain strands of HPV (usually HPV 6, 11, 16, 18), it is not recommended whilst infection is present. There is no evidence that prescribing the contraceptive pill can affect mild dyskaryosis or HPV infection. Repeat cervical smear is inappropriate given the findings of abnormal cells (mild dyskaryosis) and HPV infection, which needs to be explored further.

Public Health England. Updated cervical screening programme and colposcopy management guide; 2020.

40. D. Refer to colposcopy

Inadequate smear results occur due to an unsatisfactory specimen which the cytologist cannot interpre—for example, if there are too few cells to read or if there is too much blood on the smear. This does not mean that the smear is abnormal, but that it is unreadable. A repeat smear is usually performed after three months to reduce the risk of a further inadequate sample. However, if two consecutive smear test results are inadequate or unavailable, the patient should be referred to colposcopy after the second test. Oestrogen cream may be useful if there are signs of vaginal atrophy, but there is no evidence of that in this case.

Public Health England. Updated cervical screening programme and colposcopy management guide; 2020.

41. D. Gestational diabetes

Hyperemesis gravidarum is associated with electrolytes imbalance especially sodium and potassium, and in severe forms leading to base deficit. Lack of fluid intake or excessive fluid loss has same effect. Untreated hyperthyroidism in first trimester presents itself with severe hyperemesis and increased intestinal hurry. Chronic renal failure is associated with imbalance in potassium and phosphate levels. Gestational diabetes is usually diagnosed during second trimester as part of screening and is not associated with electrolyte imbalance.

42. E. Hormonal changes

The most important factor is hormonal change, especially high levels of progesterone. Most physiological changes are progesterone mediated. Progesterone lowers respiratory rate, leading to decreased elimination of carbon dioxide and hence lower levels of bicarbonate. Increased blood volume and renal flow tries to balance these changes.

43. B. 10–25%

The greatest risk of transmission is either with saliva or urine of infected person, and also perinatally through the ingestion of cervico-vaginal secretion. Most cases of congenital CMV are asymptomatic at birth. Only 10–25% has symptoms such as growth restriction, microcephaly, jaundice, chorioretinitis, anaemia, etc.

NHS. CMV infection. Available at: https://www.nhs.uk/conditions/cytomegalovirus-cmv

Navti O, et al. Comprehensive review and update of cytomegalovirus infection in pregnancy. *TOG* 2016;18:301–17.

44. C. She can commence the combined contraceptive pill at 6 weeks if she has risk factors for thrombosis

The FRSH UK MEC states that postpartum women without risk factors for thromboembolism should wait until 3 weeks postpartum to start combined hormonal contraception. In women who have risk factors for thromboembolism, this is extended until 6 weeks following delivery. The Mirena coil and intrauterine device is contraindicated in cases of postpartum sepsis, but otherwise may be considered within 48 hours of delivery or after 4 weeks.

FSRH UKMEC criteria; 2016, amended 2019.

45. D. Statutory ground D

The Abortion Act ground D states that, 'continuation of pregnancy would involve greater risk than termination of pregnancy, and continuation would cause injury to physical or mental health of any existing children'.

Termination of pregnancy in ground C and D can only be considered until 24 weeks.

An abortion can be carried out in ground E until term if there is a case of severe foetal abnormality.

Grounds A, B, F, and G apply to pregnancies where continuation of pregnancy involves severe risk to the woman's life or serious injury to her mental or physical health.

46. C. 0.5–2.5%

The reported incidence of epidural tap is between 0.19–3.6% and to a maximum of 12%. Furthermore the incidence depends upon the gauge of the epidural needle, lower with 18 gauge than 16 gauge.

Epidural Analgesia Network. Available at: https://www.networks.nhs.uk/nhs-networks/staffordshire-shropshire

Bateman BT, Cole N, Sun-Edelstein C, Lay CL. Post dural puncture headache. *Anesth Pain Med (Seoul)* 2023;18(2):177–89.

47. E. Sodium chloride 0.9%

This woman requires intravenous fluids as she is poorly perfused secondary to internal haemorrhage. Diuretics should not be used. Glucose infusion should be avoided as it can raise the blood glucose levels and causes fluid shift. She requires crystalloids; fluids which contain sodium (130–154 mmol/L) with an initial bolus of 500 ml given in 15 minutes.

NICE Clinical Guideline 174: Intravenous fluid therapy in adults in hospital; 2013, updated 2017.

48. E. Advance directive

Advance directive can be made by anyone over the age of 18 as regards their treatment as long as they deemed to have the capacity to make decisions following full discussion and understanding of all the relevant information. An advance directive is signed by the individual and a witness.

The decision to consult a court applies in those cases when dealing with unconscious patients or those who lack capacity.

The patient may wish to outline his/her wishes for refusing medical treatment if he/she becomes terminally ill, or if lose the ability to make decisions for him/herself. The legal document is called 'advance decision', formally called 'living will'.

'Advance refusal to treatment' is a decision; patients can make now to refuse a specific type of treatment at sometime in the future. It is only applicable if the individual loses the ability to make his/her ability to make own decision about treatment.

Mental Health Act 2007, UK. Available at: https://www.legislation.gov.uk/ukpga/2007/12/contents

49. D. Assess her Gillick competence

Gillick competence implies that a child is competent to consent to any type of treatment. She also fulfils Fraser guidelines which are specifically about contraceptive prescribing without parenteral consent. If she understands the whole procedure, its implications, and risks and benefits, then she is legally competent to sign consent. The decision rests upon the doctor who is seeing the girl whether she is Gillick competent or not.

If she is Gillick competent, then she can consent to termination without permission from her parents. Therefore, her parents or school should not be called without her consent.

Police and social services should only be involved if there are safeguarding issues.

50. C. Not to clean until DNA samples have been taken

Any significant injuries sustained should be treated with basic first aid. However, minor injuries which do not require suturing should not be cleaned because samples are required for DNA from these areas. She should be advised not to clean or wash herself, drink, or pass urine prior to the collection of all relevant samples.

Long L, Butler B. Sexual assault. *TOG* 2018;20:87–93.

Extended Matching Questions

Answers for Questions 1–5

1. C; 2. E; 3. B; 4. G; 5. L

1. C. Miller's pyramid

Miller's pyramid is used for assessing clinical competence. At the lowest level of the pyramid is knowledge (knows), followed by competence (knows how), performance (shows how), and action (does). Work-based methods of assessment target the highest level of the pyramid, whereas multiple-choice questions and simulation tests target the lower levels of the pyramid.

2. E. Objective structured clinical examination (OSCE)

Objective structured clinical examination or OSCE is an example of an assessment technique often used in a simulated environment where competencies are assessed.

3. B. Kern's 6-step framework

Kern's 6-step framework is a method used by many medical professional bodies to develop curriculums. The 6 steps used are:

Step 1: Problem identification and general needs assessment

Step 2: Targeted needs assessment

Step 3: Goals and objectives

Step 4: Educational strategies

Step 5: Implementation

Step 6: Evaluation and feedback

4. G. Outcome 2

In general, you will have a review of clinical practice annually (ARCP), who will decide based on your e-portfolio of evidence, one of the following outcomes:

Outcome 1: if the evidence provided at your ARCP is satisfactory, the panel will recommend outcome 1, indicating the successful transition to the next training year.

Outcome 2: if there are any deficiencies in your training or areas of poor performance, the panel will recommend outcome 2, which is a recommendation for targeted training to help you address these issues; if you complete this targeted training successfully, there'll be no delay to your progression to CCT or CESR(CP).

Outcome 3: if the panel identifies that you require a formal additional period of training that will extend the duration of your training programme, they will recommend an outcome 3.

Outcome 4: if there's still insufficient and sustained lack of progress despite having had up to 1 year of additional training to address concerns over progress, the panel will recommend outcome 4, which would release you from the training programme.

5. L. Pendleton's model

Pendleton's model is a way to provide feedback in education, and commonly used in medical education. It is most suitable for providing feedback for practical skills. The model follows this structure:

a) The learner describes what went well.

b) The trainer states what the learner did well.

c) The learner identifies what could be improved.

d) The trainer recognizes areas for improvement and how to achieve this.

Norcini JJ. ABC of learning and teaching in medicine: work based assessment. *BMJ* 2003;326(7392):753–5.

Kern DE. Overview: a six-step approach to curriculum development. In: Thomas PA, et al. (eds). *Curriculum development for medical education: a six-step approach*, 3rd ed. Johns Hopkins University Press, 2015; pp. 5–10.

RCOG. ARCP general information.

Qureshi NS. Giving effective feedback in medical education. *TOG* 2017;19(3):243–8.

Answers for Questions 6–10

6. J; 7. G; 8. C; 9. K; 10. B

6. J. Posterior pituitary gland

Oxytocin is a neuropeptide hormone which is produced in the hypothalamic paracentricular nucleus and released by the posterior pituitary gland. Its role is essential for lactation and labour. During labour there is an upregulation of oxytocin receptions in the uterus. It plays a role in prostaglandin synthesis, which is essential for labour progress.

7. G. L2

The ovarian arteries arise anterolaterally from the aorta just inferior to the renal arteries and superior to the inferior mesenteric artery at the level of L2. In males they are called testicular arteries. In 20% of women, they arise from the renal arteries and uncommonly may arise from adrenal, lumbar, or internal iliac arteries.

8. C. Inferior 1/3 of the rectum

The inferior mesenteric artery branches into the superior rectal artery which supplies the superior 2/3 of the rectum. The internal iliac artery branches into the middle rectal artery which supplies the inferior 1/3 of the rectum. The internal pudendal artery branches into the inferior rectal artery which supplies the anus.

9. K. Round ligament

The round ligament is a remnant of the embryonic gubernaculum. It originates at the uterine horns, and attaches to the labia majora, passing through the inguinal canal.

10. B. Cardinal ligaments

The cardinal ligaments are situated along the inferior border of the broad ligament, with the uterine arteries and veins running through them. They arise from the side of the cervix and the lateral fornix of the vagina. They provide extensive attachment on the lateral pelvic sidewall at the level of the ischial spines.

Green-top Guideline No. 5. The management of ovarian hyperstimulation syndrome; February 2016.

Answers for Questions 11–15

11. B; 12. A; 13. D; 14. I; 15. H

11. B. Cardiomyopathy

This woman has features of cardiogenic shock—including orthopnoea and signs of pulmonary congestion, which may be caused by cardiomyopathy, ischaemic heart disease, or arrhythmias.

12. A. Amniotic fluid embolism

Amniotic fluid embolism (AFE) is rare and difficult to diagnose. It is associated with a poor outcome—including maternal death—so prompt management is key. AFE should be suspected where there is acute maternal collapse with foetal compromise, cardiac arrest, cardiac arrhythmias, coagulopathy, hypotension, maternal haemorrhage, prodromal symptoms such as numbness, agitation or tingling, seizures, or shortness of breath.

13. D. Diabetic ketoacidosis

Diabetic ketoacidosis presents with an unwell patient who may complain of feeling generally unwell, blurred vision, nausea and vomiting, and hyperventilation. Ketotic breath—classically smelling like pear drops—may be noted. Initial observations may show hypotension with tachycardia and hyperventilation. An altered mental state may suggest deteriorating DKA.

14. I. Pneumonia

Viral pneumonia is more severe in pregnancy and pregnant women are particularly susceptible to chickenpox pneumonia. Symptoms include an initial dry cough, rash, fever, breathlessness, and pleuritic pain. Clinical signs include purulent sputum, coarse crackles on auscultation, and signs of consolidation.

15. H. Placental abruption

The main issue here is the presentation of severe constant lower abdominal pain with a background history of a fall. The examination findings and foetal heart rate point towards a diagnosis of placental abruption.

Burns R, Dent K. *ALSG: managing medical and obstetric emergencies and trauma: a practical approach*, 4th ed. Oxford: Wiley-Blackwell; 2022.

Nelson-Piercy C. *Obstetric medicine*, 6th ed. Boca Raton: CRC Press; 2020.

RCOG Green-top Guideline 13. Chickenpox in pregnancy; 2015.

Answers for Questions 16–20

16. E; 17 F; 18 G; 19. I; 20. L

16. E. Failure to visualize the uterine cavity

Here, the patient has had multiple operations to her uterus. Specifically, a uterine ablation and transcervical resection of fibroids along with her raised BMI may make it more difficult to enter and visualize the uterine cavity.

17. F. Faecal or flatus incontinence

The main risk associated with a third or fourth-degree perineal tears is faecal or flatus incontinence.

18. G. Haemorrhage requiring blood transfusion

This is the most common serious risk associated with abdominal hysterectomy for benign conditions, occurring in 23 women in every 1,000 (common). This is more common than damage to the bladder and/or ureter (7 women in every 1,000) or injury to the bowel (4 in every 10,000 women). 7 in every 1,000 women require a return to theatre because of bleeding or wound dehiscence.

19. I. Intrauterine adhesions

Intrauterine adhesions were reported in 3–38% of miscarriages, with a risk of 16–18% in cases of surgical evacuation, ranging in severity and extent. The frequency and severity of intrauterine adhesions are proportional to the number of surgical evacuation procedures performed.

20. L. Urinary incontinence

Urinary incontinence occurring over a year after birth occurs in about 1 in 4 women following a planned caesarean section and is seen in about 1 in 2 women following a planned vaginal birth. However, there is an associated risk of urinary tract injury of about in per 1,000 women, which is not seen with a planned vaginal birth.

Burns R, Dent K. *ALSG: managing medical and obstetric emergencies and trauma: a practical approach*, 4th ed. Oxford: Wiley-Blackwell; 2022.

RCOG Consent Advice No 4. Abdominal hysterectomy for benign conditions; 2009.

RCOG Consent Advice No 10. Surgical managerment of miscarriage and removal of persistent placental or fetal remains; 2018.

Answers for Questions 21–25

21. C; 22. E; 23. F; 24. A; 25. G

21. C. CT abdomen and pelvis

There is a likely possibility of uterine perforation and bowel injury. Therefore, a CT scan should be arranged.

22. E. CT urogram

There is a strong possibility of ureteric injury presenting as loin pain. Constipation may be secondary to excessive use of analgesics.

23. F. Cystogram

There is a high possibility of vesico-vaginal fistula

24. A. Bladder scan

It is possible that the patient is not well perfused. Bladder scan in the ward will show if there is any issue either with the catheter (full bladder but not draining) or an empty bladder which would require a different line of approach (fluid challenge test first, then CT urogram if urinary tract injury is being suspected).

25. G. Intermittent self-catheterization

It is not uncommon to have minor postoperative voiding difficulties following this procedure. Rather than resting the bladder, intermittent catheterization is considered a better approach.

Answers for Questions 26–30

26. I; 27. D; 28. A; 29. K; 30. F

26. I. No treatment

A history of varicose veins is not an indication for LMWH prophylaxis.

27. D. Close surveillance antenatally and prophylactic LMWH postnatally for 6 weeks

Risk identification should be made by using the RCOG recommendation, and management should be planned. As she has at least one risk factor identified, she should be closely observed during pregnancy, and post-partum prophylaxis be provided.

Any pregnant woman with two or more risk factors should be assessed for prophylaxis both antenatally and postnatally individually.

RCOG Green-top Guideline No 37a. Reducing the risk of thromboembolism during pregnancy and the puerperium; 2015.

28. A. Change to heparinoid danaparoid sodium

As LMWH has led to thrombocytopenia, she should be changed over to heparinoid danaparoid sodium during antenatal period. She can be managed with warfarin postnatally.

29. K. Prophylactic LMWH antenatally and postnatally for 6 weeks

She should be offered prophylaxis with LMWH and also advised to use graduated elastic compression stockings during post-partum for 6–12 weeks.

30. F. Commence prophylactic LMWH

Because of her previous history of deep venous thrombosis, she should be commenced on LMWH as early as possible. She has no other identifiable risk factors. LMWH should be continued during pregnancy and continued for six weeks postnatally.

Answers to Questions 31–35

31. B; 32. F; 33. D; 34. L; 35. M

31. B. Bowel injury

The most likely diagnosis in this case is injury to the small bowel, which could have been adherent to the anterior abdominal wall with omental bands following her previous pelvic surgery.

32. F. Injury to internal iliac vessel

This patient has a low BMI and hence the anterior abdominal wall is very thin. In such patients, ideally Hassan's open technique should be used to introduce blunt trocar through the umbilicus for laparoscopy. A sudden drop in blood pressure is due to Verres needle injury to one of the branches of the internal iliac artery. It is a retroperitoneal structure,; extravasations of blood are in the retroperitoneal space and is not visible. This interrupts blood supply to the bowel and gives a picture of under perfusion.

33. D. Inferior epigastric vessel injury

Once the pneumoperineum has been created, and the laparoscope has been introduced, the lateral trocar should be introduced under direct vision. It is important to clearly identify the descending inferior epigastric artery by its anatomical landmarks or shining light against the anterior abdominal wall. Furthermore, the trocar should be introduced vertically without any displacement of tissues in the anterior abdominal wall.

34. L. Ureteric injury

Pelvic endometriosis is associated with extensive fibrosis, therefore tissue dissection is often challenging. Ovarian endometrioma and ovary are quite often densely adherent to the lateral pelvic wall and the underlying ureter. Therefore, the ureter is at risk of either crushing injury at the time of surgery or may present as ischaemic injury a few weeks later on. This is a case of ureteric injury incurred at the time of surgery. Urine is draining into the pelvic cavity, hence elevated levels of urea and free fluid in the pelvis. Preoperative retrograde ureteric stenting should be considered in these cases.

35. M. Uterine perforation

In this case, the most likely diagnosis is perforation of the uterus, which is a recognized complication of this procedure. Other differential diagnoses include fluid overload and postoperative pain.

Answers to Questions 36–40

36. L; 37. B; 38. B; 39. I; 40. E

36. L. Penicillin and probiotics vaginally

Bacterial vaginosis (BV) is the most common cause of vaginal discharge caused by *Gardnerella vaginalis*. Presence of Group B Strep Agalactiae, which is a Gram-positive bacterium, lowers the lactobacilli and creates inflammatory conditions. In this patient, antibiotics should be given to treat GBS and probiotics be given vaginally to change vaginal pH while for BV, vaginal clindamycin and metronidazole may be prescribed.

37. B. Canesten vaginally and oral itraconazole

Investigations should exclude host factors such as diabetes, immunosuppression, use of antibiotics, and iron deficiency anaemia, etc. Differential diagnosis should include dermatitis, eczema, lichen sclerosis, BV, and vulvodynia. As she has had more than three episodes of candidiasis, she should be treated with a prolonged course for six months.

38. B. Flucloxacillin

This is a Bartholin's inflamed cyst and should be initially treated with antibiotics. STI screening should also be carried out.

39. I. Ofloxacin and metronidazole

This is a case of acute inflammatory pelvic infection. The vaginal discharge description is more suggestive of bacterial vaginosis. While bloods and swabs are being sent, she will need treatment with broad-spectrum antibiotics.

40. E. Erythromycin

The clinical features of this case are suggestive of infection with chlamydia trachomatis. Infection primarily occurs through penetrative sexual intercourse. The cervix is infected in over 75% cases and the urethra in 50–60% cases. If left untreated, it will lead to ascending infection within pelvic organs.

Bitzer J, Mahmood T (eds). *Handbook of contraception and sexual reproductive health.* Cambridge: Cambridge University Press; 2022.

Answers for Questions 41–50

41. A; 42. N; 43. G; 44. K; 45. H

41. A. Consent by patient

Consent by the patient is required if she is regarded as Gillick competent. Parental consent is not required and neither court of law's involvement is necessary. Consent can be written or verbal as long as the patient fully understands the reason for surgery, risks, and benefits, and what the surgery entails.

42. N. Wishes of mother/parents needs to be respected

She has the right to decline post-mortem as long she understands its implication. Court action has no place in this case. Any other alternative investigations other than post-mortem require the mother's consent.

43. G. No registration of stillbirth required

As this baby died at 18 weeks gestation (<24 weeks which is regarded as the stage of viability in law), there is no need to register it as stillbirth.

44. K. Register as neonatal death

This baby has shown signs of life, and therefore should be registered as neonatal death irrespective of weight or gestational age.

45. H. Not to proceed with the surgery

As this is a benign cyst, no further surgery should be carried out. Partner's consent has no legal validity.

RCOG. Clinical governance advice No. 6. Obtaining valid consent; 2015.

Answers to Questions 46–50

46. B; 47. E; 48. C; 49. L; 50. J

46. B. Femoral nerve

Femoral neuropathy commonly occurs following compression of the nerve against the pelvic side wall, especially when deep retractor blades are used for lateral placement in difficult cases of pelvic surgery.

47. E. Ileo-inguinal nerve

Injury to the ileo-inguinal nerve is typically caused by suture entrapment at the lateral border of the low transverse incision, which has been extended beyond the lateral border of the rectus abdominus muscle.

48. C. Genitofemoral nerve

The genitofemoral nerve makes its way through the psoas muscle, which attaches the spine to the top of the hips on both sides. It branches into the genital and femoral nerves just above the inguinal ligament. The genital branch innervates the labia majora and mons pubis. Some medical conditions can also lead to peripheral neuropathy. The nerve can also be damaged during lymph node dissection for uterine, ovarian, or bladder cancer surgery, or when a large mass is removed during pelvic surgery.

49. L. Sciatic nerve

Risk factors for sciatic nerve injury include obesity, prolonged sitting, age-related changes in the spine such as herniated discs and bone spurs, occupations carrying heavy loads and even driving vehicles for long periods, and uncontrolled diabetes. It can also present during pregnancy because of hormonal changes, shifting forward of the mother's centre of gravity, pressure of the growing uterus, and the baby's position causing pressure on the nerve.

50. J. Pudendal nerve

The pudendal nerve arises from S2, S3, and S4. It enters the perineum via the lesser sciatic foramen running in the pudendal canal. It supplies sensory branches to the external genitalia and motor supply to the pelvic muscles and external anal sphincter. Therefore, the pudendal nerve block is ideal for instrumental deliveries.

INDEX OF QUESTIONS BY RCOG MODULE

This table shows each RGOC module and the Paper and relevant question(s) which address those topics.

S = SBA questions

E = EMQ questions

Knowledge area	Paper 1	Paper 2	Paper 3	Paper 4	Paper 5	Paper 6
Clinical skills		S2, S7, S32		S14	S32, S45	S10, S11, S13, S14, S16, S47, S48, S49, S50
		E21–E25	E21–E25, E31–E35	E46–E50		
Teaching and research	S15	S13, S29, S41	S24	S25	S1	S17, S18, S19, S20
		E43–E47	E36–E40	E36–E40		E1–E5
Core surgical skills		S1, S4, S18, S40	S3, S10	S35, S36, S44, S50		S1, S2, S4, S5, S6, S7, S8, S9, S12, S15, S22, S29, S46
					E10–E14	E6–E10, E16–E20, E31–E35, E41–E45, E46–E50
Postoperative care		E32, E48–E50			S35, S48	S34
						E21–E25
Antenatal care	S14, S22, S23, S26, S28, S36, S39, S44	S8, S19, S26, S36, S38	S7, S13, S19, S22, S30, S31, S41, S43, S46	S6, S16, S17, S20, S23, S38, S41	S9, S12, S16, S21, S23, S27, S29, S38, S49	S3, S30
	E10			E31–E35	E26, E27	E26–E30
Maternal medicine	S1, S7, S20, S31, S34, S41, S43	S9, S12, S15, S17, S21, S27, S30, S34, S45, S47	S5, S15, S27, S32	S4, S19, S28, S32, S39, S42, S43, S48, S30	S3, S4, S6, S14, S17, S20, S25, S34, S37	S24, S41, S42, S43
	E1–5, E7	E6–E10, E11–E15	E1–E5, E6–E10, E21–E25		E21–E25, E36–E40	E11–E15
Management of labour	S32,	S10, S31	S17, S37, S47	S8, S21, S29		S10, S25, S26
	E13			E1, E2, E4, E5		

Knowledge area	Paper 1	Paper 2	Paper 3	Paper 4	Paper 5	Paper 6
Management of delivery	S5, S16	S4, S44	S28, S44	S11, S34		S21, S27
	E6, E11, E12, E14, E15			E3	E28–E30	
Postpartum problems	S6, S27, S42	S23, S39, S49	S11, S26	S13, S24		S23, S31, S32, S44
	E8, E9		E26–E30		E15–E20	
Gynaecological problems	S3, S9, S21, S37, S45, S48	S5, S11, S16, S20, S35, S42, S46, S48	S14, S34, S38, S49	S5, S22, S30, S46	S8, S18, S36, S43	
	E16, E17	E37–E42	E46–E50	E11–E15, E21–E25, E26–E30	E1–E5, E33–E35, E46–E50	
Subfertility	S12, S24, S40	S25, S37, S50	S16, S39, S45	S9, S10, S18	S10, S22	S28
		E1–E5, E16–E20	E42–E45		E6–E9, E31, E32	
Sexual and reproductive health	S8, S17, S18, S30	S3,	S21, S33, S42	S3, S15, S26, S40, S45, S49	S11, S15, S33, S39, S41, S46	S33, S45
	E41–E47	E26–E30	E11–E15			E36–E40
Early pregnancy care	S4, S10, S13, S19, S29	S43	S9, S18, S20, S29, S40	S47	S28	
	E20, E21–25, E26–30, E36, E37		E41	E6–E10		
Gynaecological oncology	S2, S11, S25, S33, S35, S46, S49	S14, S22, S24, S28	S6, S12, S23, S25, S35, S48	S12, S27, S31, S33, S37	S2, S7, S13, S19, S24, S31, S40, S42, S47, S50	S35, S36, S37, S38, S39, S40
	E18, E19, E31	E31–E36	E16–E20			
Urogynaecology & pelvic floor problems	S38, S47, S50	S33	S36, S50	S7	S26, S44	
	E33–E35, E38–E30	E48–E50		E16–E20, E41–E45	E41–E45	

INDEX

For the benefit of digital users, indexed terms that span two pages (e.g., 52–53) may, on occasion, appear on only one of those pages.